BODY BAR

133 Moves for Full-Body Fitness

Gregg Cook & Fatima d'Almeida-Cook

Foreword by Sherry Catlin

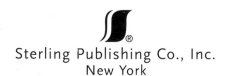
Sterling Publishing Co., Inc.
New York

If you are not used to exercising, are pregnant, or have any other medical condition, please check with your doctor before beginning any form of exercise.

Library of Congress Cataloging-in-Publication Data

Cook, Gregg.
    Body bar : 133 moves for full-body fitness / Gregg Cook and Fatima d'Almeida-Cook ; foreword by Sherry Catlin.
        p. cm.
    Includes index.
    ISBN-13: 978-1-4027-3190-7
    ISBN-10: 1-4027-3190-6
    1. Physical fitness—Equipment and supplies.   I. D'Almeida-Cook, Fatima. II. Title.
    GV543.C66 2006
    613.7'170284—dc22

                                                                2006025470

10 9 8 7 6 5 4 3 2 1

Published by Sterling Publishing Co., Inc.
387 Park Avenue South, New York, NY 10016
© 2006 by Gregg Cook and Fatima d'Almeida-Cook
Distributed in Canada by Sterling Publishing
c/o Canadian Manda Group, 165 Dufferin Street
Toronto, Ontario, Canada M6K 3H6
Distributed in the United Kingdom by GMC Distribution Services
Castle Place, 166 High Street, Lewes, East Sussex, England BN7 1XU
Distributed in Australia by Capricorn Link (Australia) Pty. Ltd.
P.O. Box 704, Windsor, NSW 2756, Australia

Manufactured in China
All rights reserved

Sterling ISBN-13:978-1-4027-3190-7
        ISBN-10:1-4027-3190-6

For information about custom editions, special sales, premium and corporate purchases, please contact Sterling Special Sales Department at 800-805-5489 or specialsales@sterlingpub.com.

Contents

Foreword

To most people, how to get in shape is a complete mystery. We are bombarded from every direction with new fitness products, crazy diets, and wild workouts; the options are endless, overwhelming, and often paralyzing. Yard sales, eBay, and sidewalks on trash day are filled with the dusty remains of little-used or useless exercise equipment that was just too big, too complicated, too difficult, or too "not right for me." Still, hope is alive and millions are spent on the new "new" thing that will finally flatten your belly, carve your thighs, or melt away those last 20 pounds.

Well, now you can save your money and your floor space. The *Body Bar* book and one simple Body Bar will provide enough exercises and workouts to get or keep your body looking and feeling great. Gregg Cook is a seasoned and consummate fitness professional who brings a fresh perspective and innovative approach to this simple, classic tool. His creative workouts focus on developing a body that has usable strength, functional mobility, and the endurance to move through life with ease and grace. Fatima's down-to-earth and lighthearted narrative takes the mystery out of strength training and creates a simple, easy-to-follow guide to fitness for every age and every body.

So, grab a Body Bar . . . yes, just one. One piece, no assembly required. Start light; Gregg's workouts show that it's not about how much weight you lift, but about what you do with that weight. Learn the proper form and technique in the beginning of the book and you're ready to go.

If you are new to the Body Bar or to exercise, don't worry; Gregg will show you just what to do. The handbook offers a tremendous variety and range of workouts that are safe, effective, and fun. Even experienced weekend warriors, athletes, and trainers will find them comprehensive and cutting-edge.

No time? Open the handbook and do one exercise. It all adds up. The commercials of your favorite nighttime TV show add up to another 20 minutes, so keep your Body Bar close at hand—and use it!

Life is complicated . . . fitness should be simple. So just move more, eat less, and lift weight. Make that weight a Body Bar—it doesn't get much simpler than that.

Sherry Catlin
IDEA International 2004 Program Director of the Year
President, Body Bar Systems
sherry.catlin@verizon.net

Introduction

What It Is

The Body Bar could arguably be one of the most versatile and simply effective pieces of fitness equipment on the market today. It is used as a training tool in countless ways all over the world. Nowadays, Body Bars are used at gyms, on the training floor, as well as in group fitness classes ranging from circuit and interval classes to kickboxing classes, sports conditioning classes, and Pilates and yoga-based classes. You can also find Body Bars at schools and universities, parks and recreation centers, retirement communities, spas, and military bases. Given its versatility and simplicity of storage and use, it is likely that if you took a peek into your next-door neighbor's closet, you would find a Body Bar.

A Body Bar is a solid piece of steel sheathed in a durable and cushiony-soft rubber. There are sixteen different Body Bar variations. They vary in both weight and length, so that you will have no problem finding a bar that will work for you whether you are a complete novice or an experienced fitness authority. The bars are capped on both ends with brightly colored indicators. These indicators clearly display the weight of each bar so that there is no guesswork involved in choosing the appropriate one.

In order to achieve all that is demanded of us, we must regard ourselves as greater than we are.

—Johann Wolfgang von Goethe

Wonder Bar

Wondering . . . what they were thinking when they named the product the "Body Bar"? It's kind of perfect, isn't it? Brilliant marketing, if you ask us. It sounds rather intriguing; perhaps the name of the latest happy hour concept. Well, the Body Bar is not consumable but absolutely delicious to use nonetheless. With all the new things and different exercises you will learn from using this book, you will be intoxicated with excitement and energy for a new Body Bar workout every day (maybe even two or three times a day). Even better, with the Body Bar, there is no chance of suffering the often-experienced morning-after-happy-hour maladies. Instead you will be filled with a distinct feeling of a strong, lasting, and very bearable lightness of being . . . and a fuller piggy bank to boot.

The Body Bar is available in all the varieties listed below.

Mini Bars
Length: 2 feet
Weight: 2, 4, 6, 9, or 12 pounds

Petite Bars
Length: 3 feet
Weight: 3, 6, or 9 pounds

Classic Bars
Length: 4 feet
Weight: 4, 9, 12, 15, 18, or 24 pounds

Big and Tall Bars
Length: 5 feet
Weight: 30 pounds

Giant Bars
Length: 6 feet
Weight: 36 pounds

The Man Behind the Bar

The Body Bar was founded by Arno P. Niemand and has been manufactured in the United States since 1987. It all began in New York City, when trainer Steve Kelly, an Olympic kayaker, brought some of his kayaking training to Arno's sessions. They used steel bars that were rough on the hands—as well as every other surface they came in contact with—but were exceptionally versatile. Arno found that he was getting an amazing workout with this tool and was struck with the ingenious idea that he wanted to share it with the world. The first Body Bar and the dawn of a new era in fitness came shortly after.

Why the Body Bar Is So Great

The biggest difference between the Body Bar and other types of strength-training equipment such as dumbbells and plate-loaded bars is in the distribution of weight. The Body Bar is a free weight that has evenly distributed weight throughout. What does this mean? There are no attachments needed and no loose parts. There is no danger that the bar will tilt to one side and fall over dramatically. The classic Body Bar is 4 feet long. This length is ideal (for most people) for standing the bar vertically beside you as a tool to help support you as you balance. Because the bars are straight and long, they can also be used as a handy device to help assess alignment with certain exercises. (We'll show you how.) Traditional plate-loaded bars are too long and too heavy to be used in either of these ways.

The rubber padding cleverly encasing the steel bar allows you to focus on the body part intended, not the tough and unattractive calluses forming on the palms of your hands. It provides a comfortable, safe, and slip-free gripping surface, so the bar is less likely to slip out of your hands and onto your foot, or someone else's for that matter.

Body Bars are easy to hide away. They are the perfect piece of equipment to have anywhere, even if your space is limited. They are neat and compact, and a simple corner in your closet provides enough space to store them. (Don't let this be an excuse for never taking your Body Bars out!)

Body Bars are simple to use. For all those who are challenged by the mere thought of piecing together a puzzle, the Body Bar is the picture of fitness utopia. There is no assembly required.

Body Bars are a resourceful investment. In this book, you will no doubt be able to find at least one or several Body Bar workouts you will thrive on. We encourage you to use what you learn in this book to create your own personalized workout as well. Body Bars are adaptable to almost any type of training and will complement almost any type of equipment you may currently own or use. Because there are so many weight and length options available, Body Bars can be used as the sole tool for a workout, as well as in conjunction with other pieces of equipment such as a medicine ball, Swiss ball, Bosu, Urban Rebounder, step, stretching straps, and bands. The options are virtually limitless.

Reach for a Body Bar instead of a chocolate bar. Try storing your Body Bars in the pantry, right next to the unhealthy snacks.

Strength Training: The Meaning of It

The importance of adding strength training to a workout repertoire is becoming increasingly acknowledged. So, what does strength training mean, exactly? Don't think that it has anything to do with the half-naked, lubed-up, and über-tanned bodybuilders you see on

Check out www.bodybars.com, the official Body Bar Web site. There you will be able to purchase any or all of the Body Bars you could possibly want, as well as creative and innovative videos you can use to help guide you along visually and keep your workouts interesting. There are more than 30 Body Bar workouts on DVD available on the market today.

late-night cable. Strength training is simply the disciplined addition of weight or resistance to exercises in order to train your muscles to have the capacity to handle more. In other words, you will be training your muscles to become stronger. As with anything else, the more you do something, the better you get at it, and the less of a challenge it becomes. As you practice, your body adapts to the weights or resistance, and you in turn are able to handle more.

Why We Do It

So, why train at all? Why voluntarily elect to squeeze a vigorous workout into your already overflowing schedule? Aren't we all trying to simplify our lives, which are already so replete with unjustifiable and superfluous nuisances? What makes it all worth it? There are several inarguably flawless answers to this question. Here are a few of our favorites in order of increasing significance.

The most obvious and simplest is wrapped up in one word: vanity. That we all want to look good is no enigmatic bit of information. Adding training to your lifestyle will help you build muscle and burn calories quicker, and thus, you will be working your way toward the slim and trim figure you've always dreamed of.

Another answer, even better in our opinion, is that by training your body, you will become stronger and healthier. Being stronger in your workouts translates into being stronger in your life . . . being able to pick up a bag of groceries, your five-year-old child, your twelve-year-old child. You will be a frustrating thorn in the side of aging and its relentless attempts to slow you down. Loads of money and materialistic success will be of no use to you if you are physically consumed with too many aches and pains to enjoy them. Strength training will earn you stronger muscles, including the most important muscle of all, your heart, and as a result, will lessen your chances of developing heart disease. Your joints will be well supported and your posture will be improved. You will have strong bones, decreasing your risk of osteoporosis, you will increase your metabolism and calorie burning during resistance training, and all in all, you will increase fat loss. You will

Personally, we love using the Body Bar . . . for personal training sessions. One or two Body Bars are enough for a full-body workout. They are easy to use, even in small spaces. Living in New York City, where space is limited, we find that this feature is essential. Body Bars are also easy to transport and add variety to a workout. As we all know, variety is the spice of life—this applies to workout life as well!

be able to function more freely and independently in life, and you will experience fewer aches and pains well into your golden years.

The ultimate, all-encompassing, and most important answer to the question of why we train lies in the fact that our minds, bodies, and spirits are completely interconnected. We do whatever it takes to look good in order to feel good, in an attempt to move toward the experience of happiness. The secret is this: Something easily attained—perhaps given to you in the form of a "magic pill"—does not come with the same sense of fulfillment as it would, had it been earned through hard work and discipline. This is true of anything in life. The act of taking control of your body and working toward becoming stronger, leaner, and healthier overall will bring results that are valuable psychologically, emotionally, and physically. What makes life worthwhile is actually experiencing it. In the same sense, experience your body and its phenomenal ability to move. Make the most of it. Challenge it. Really, it is all you've got with absolute certainty and within your control. Treat it right. Training it to be the best it can be is a wonderful way of cherishing it.

What to Do with This Book

Our first line of business is to initiate you into working out. We have put together a list of "Bar Basics" comprised of instructions and precautions partially geared toward using the Body Bar and this book, but essentially for any workout regimen.

Chapter 1, "The Breakdown," is a photographic and descriptive how-to for performing exercises with the Body Bar. For each exercise, we tell you what muscles you will be working ("The Focus"), how to set up ("The Setup"), and how to do the exercise ("The Move"). In addition, we share ways to modify the exercises to suit your fitness level (or feeling of the day), as well as some extra tips. The exercises are separated into body parts from biggest muscle group (lower body) to smallest (triceps, biceps). We have also included a section for core, multitask exercises, which link two or more moves to create one "functional movement," and a section for plyometric, quickness, and agility exercises.

Chapter 2, "The Workouts," begins with a list of exercises we call "the Fundamentals." You should be familiar with them in order to perform any of the workouts. They are the starting point. From there

As our friend Tom likes to say, as a society, we are unanimously in pursuit of immortality. Training will bring you one step closer.

As with any new exercise, start with a light and manageable bar. Once you become comfortable with the movement and find the exercise becoming easy to handle, you can try moving to a heavier bar. Keep in mind that more does not mean better. What is most important is not the weight of the bar you use, it is your ability to use the bar creatively and effectively with good form and technique.

you will be ready to rock and roll. We show you how to turn the individual exercises into balanced training sessions with a series of 10- to 40-minute workouts ranging from beginner level to intermediate to advanced.

Chapter 3, "The Home Stretch," shows you a few ways to stretch some of the most common tight spots.

To guarantee a friendly and welcoming Body Bar experience, we suggest that you begin with the Fundamentals and follow them with the beginner workouts. Once those exercises start feeling fuzzy-just-out-of-the-dryer comfortable to you, you are ready to move on. Ease yourself into the next step. Try combining beginner workouts with intermediate and advanced workouts. When you begin to feel like an old pro, try mixing it up in any random way you want.

Wonder Bar

Wondering . . . how to make your workout more challenging? Go for a heavier weight, or take a shorter break in between exercises, or combine both for a real challenge.

Bar Basics

The Props

Most of the exercises in this book require the use of only your Body Bar(s). Some exercises are most effectively done with the use of some sort of bench, step, platform, or Bosu. For some moves you can even use the steps of a staircase if you have nothing else. Use one step if you are a beginner. Use two if you are more advanced. If you're no longer challenged by two steps of your staircase, your stairs may be limiting and we suggest that you buy one of the alternative type stairs.

Wonder Bar

Wondering . . . what a Bosu is? It is an air-filled dome that can be used both dome side up and platform side up. Because of its unstable surface, it will add a balance challenge to your workout. (See www.bosu.com.) Use it as a more difficult alternative to a traditional platform.

It is also handy to have an exercise mat, yoga mat, towel, or blanket for exercises that require you to get down on the floor. Use whatever you have available that is comfortable to you.

The Dress Code

What should you wear? Location is the key to this question. Depending on whether you are working out in public or in private, our words of advice vary. Any time you are going to be publicly visible, we strongly discourage the birthday suit. In fact, we strictly forbid it. In private, just about anything goes, including nothing. Do as you wish, but if you are working out publicly or if you privately decide to wear something, make sure it is comfortable. You want to be able to move dynamically and easily but not have too much excess fabric draping over you. You should be able to bend down, raise your legs in the air, twist and turn, raise your arms, and lie on your back or your belly without tripping or getting caught in anything. Beware of sports bras that are decorated with cumbersome contraptions. Heavy hardware, such as zippers and buttons, and even simple knots can sometimes be unpleasantly intruding. (Remember the children's story the "Princess and the Pea"?)

Snug-fitting clothing made from stretchy but breathable fabrics works very well. In this day and age, there are many amazing technical fabrics available for working out. Some of our favorites include Lycra, Supplex, Coolmax, and Dri-FIT. Lycra and Supplex will

We all have different capacities for sweating. There is nothing wrong with generating sweat, whether in the form of tiny beads budding on your forehead or a small pond slowly rising around you. Sweating is the body's natural cooling system, with an added pore-cleaning bonus. That said, what could be more awkward and repugnant than slipping and falling in a pool of sweat, especially someone else's? Do not be the cause of your own or someone else's demise. Keep the area you are working in dry. Have a towel handy!

Wonder Bar

Wondering . . . how you know whether the bar you are using for a particular exercise is too light or too heavy? Begin with a weight that you can manage with good form. Worry about getting the moves right first. As a general guideline, you should be able to do a minimum of 10 to 15 repetitions with the bar you are using. If you can't, switch to a lighter bar. If you have several different bars available to you, don't be afraid to use a variety of them. Try different bars for different exercises. Consider increasing the weight only once you have perfected your form.

give a garment stretch and allow you to move freely and comfortably within it. Coolmax and Dri-FIT work in a vacuumlike fashion, pulling moisture away from your body, to the surface layer of the garment, allowing the moisture to evaporate and the garment to dry quickly. These fibers will allow you to move without restraint, while keeping you drier and cooler throughout your workout.

Regarding footwear, again, the criteria are different for the public and private milieus. Most public facilities, including all gyms, require you to wear some sort of closed-toe training shoe. The reason for this is safety. The descent of an accidentally dropped weight on your naked little toe (or your neighbor's), even if it is one of the featherweight two-pounders, can be quite painful and is a lawsuit waiting to happen. When using the Body Bar, any type of training shoe will work; however, some of the exercises in this book require a certain amount of lateral movement. For this we recommend that you wear a shoe that supports you with a wider base such as a cross trainer.

If you're training privately, a cross-training shoe is great as well, but essentially, footwear is optional. Remember to be careful. Dropping something on your foot at home may not be as embarrassing as doing it in the gym but will be equally painful. When choosing footwear for the home workout, for obvious reasons don't opt for a stiletto. Also

Protect yourself from accidentally exposing anything you may otherwise save for doctors and lovers. Wear the proper undergarments. Sports bras are essential. Wear them alone or under your T-shirts and tank tops. Some type of supportive undergarment, such as compression shorts, is mandatory under your looser shorts. They will hold you together nicely and will make your workout more comfortable. Your workout neighbors will appreciate this as well.

stay away from any other type of shoe that may allow the accidental escape of your feet, that is, flip-flops or fuzzy slippers.

How do you know what weight and how many bars to start out with? One Body Bar to start is absolutely fine. In general, if habitual exercise has already infused its way into your life, a 12-pound bar is probably a good weight to start out with. If you are not acclimated to working out and are just getting started, try a 9-pound bar. We like having two different weights available, a heavier bar and a lighter bar. Because certain body parts are stronger than others, we are able to get a more specific and thorough workout with the ability to alternate between the weights.

Avoid a sudden up-close and personal encounter with your floor. If you are working out in a small space, be conscious of where you place the Body Bars you are not using. Try to keep them far enough away from your working space so that you don't accidentally stumble over one.

Stay in control at all times, and by this we don't just mean control your temper. Don't yank and jerk the Body Bar (or your own body, for that matter) around. Work to keep your movements slow and controlled throughout each exercise . . . as you lift, as you lower, as you extend, as you contract, and as you hold steady.

The Alignment of Your Body

Body alignment is of paramount importance in any form of exercise. When you stand, on either one foot or both feet, be sure to keep your weight evenly distributed. In other words, don't allow your feet to turn inward or outward. Your joints should always be properly

> Exercise is only as beneficial as the posture in which you perform it.
>
> —Matthias Alexander

Wonder Bar

Wondering . . . what the definition of core is? Imagine your body, minus your arms and legs. That is your core. It is made up of all the muscles that support your spine, including your neck. All movement affects and is affected by your core. By strengthening your core you are creating support for all your body's movements in life.

aligned. For most exercises, your hips, knees, and toes should always face the same direction. You also don't want to lean forward and on the balls of your feet, or lean back and completely on your heels. Feel every part of your feet on the floor—each of your toes, your heels, and the balls of your feet.

Contract your abdominals by pulling your navel in toward your spine. This will help keep your pelvis in a neutral position and will protect your lower back. An easy way to think of this is to imagine wearing a corset.

Roll your shoulders down and back. This should give your chest a lifted and open feeling. Keep your neck long. Imagine lifting out from the top of your head. Keep your knees soft. Never lock any of your joints. Keep your wrists straight and strong.

There is a simple way to make sure that you are holding the Body Bar evenly across your shoulders and that you are standing up straight and not using one side of your body more than the other. Take a look at yourself in the mirror. Take note of your shoulders. Both sides should be completely level. Make the proper adjustments before beginning an exercise.

To avoid poor form, when holding the bar on your shoulders, avoid draping your arms over the bar like a scarecrow. You'll want to make sure that you avoid having a curved back, shoulders rolling forward,

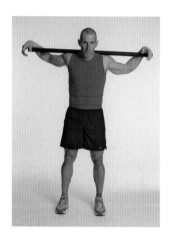

Scarecrow

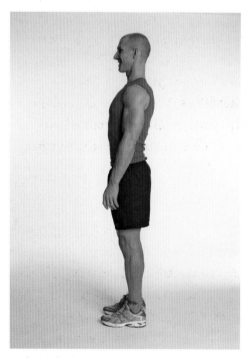

Natural Standing Position

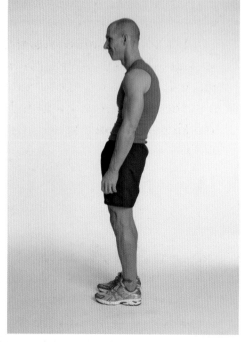

Bad Form

and neck jutting out, as the illustration on this page shows. Not so attractive, is it?

Many of the exercises in this book will begin in a Natural Standing Position. We call it this because it is a healthy posture, keeping the spine in neutral alignment. With practice, it should feel natural. Here is how to achieve this posture: Stand with your feet between hip- and shoulder-width apart; your toes pointed straight ahead (your hips, knees, and toes should create a straight line); your navel pulled in toward your spine; your chest lifted; and your shoulders down and back. Keep your weight evenly distributed between both feet, over your ankles.

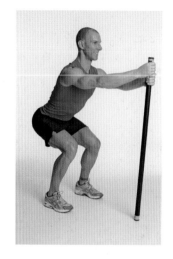

The Progression

When using the Body Bar for most leg exercises and some of the more dynamic exercises we show you, there are three different ways you can hold the bar. We have listed them below in order of difficulty, from beginner to advanced.

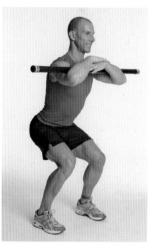

1. Vertically—Let the Body Bar be your staff, a tool to help you maintain your balance.
2. Cradled in your arms—Holding the bar this way will add weight to the movement. The bar should be held securely in your arms. In this position, the Body Bar adds weight to the front of your body. It will challenge your core significantly while you work.
3. On your shoulders—With the bar resting on your trapezius muscle (the meatier part of your shoulders, below the neck), hold on to the bar with an overhand grip, your hands slightly wider than shoulder width apart. Keep your elbows directly under your hands.

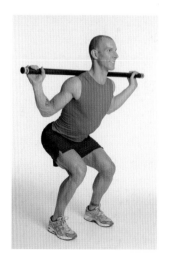

The Extras

▥ Don't forget to warm up before getting into the main part of your workout. Warm muscles will minimize the risk of injury.
▥ Don't forget to stretch after your workout or after an exercise. This is the best time to stretch, not before your muscles are warm.
▥ Don't forget to breathe. Although forgetting to breathe is unusual

while performing everyday activities, suffering a breathing blank-out during exercise is quite common. Make it a habit to breathe deeply and freely. Use your breath to your advantage. Here is the general exercise-breathing rule: Breathe in through your nose deep into your belly before the movement; breathe out through your nose or mouth during the movement.

■ Don't forget to keep hydrated . . . drink water. While you don't want to fill your belly up so much that it sounds like an ocean while you are working out, don't wait until you are fully parched to take a sip of water. Take little sips throughout your workout. Keep your water bottle handy. For an extra boost of energy in our workouts and quicker recovery, we add Amino Vital to our water. For more information, see www.amino-vital.com. (It tastes great too!)

The Breakdown

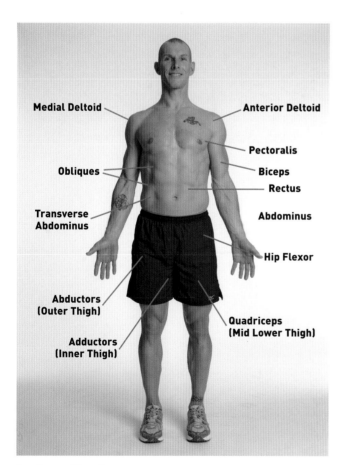

Medial Deltoid
Anterior Deltoid
Pectoralis
Obliques
Biceps
Rectus
Transverse Abdominus
Abdominus
Hip Flexor
Abductors (Outer Thigh)
Adductors (Inner Thigh)
Quadriceps (Mid Lower Thigh)

Anatomy Front

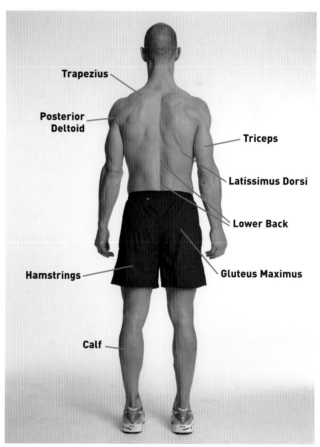

Trapezius
Posterior Deltoid
Triceps
Latissimus Dorsi
Lower Back
Hamstrings
Gluteus Maximus
Calf

Anatomy Rear

Wonder Bar

Wondering . . . what it feels like to engage your shoulder blades into your back? Try this: With your chin off your chest, focus on something straight ahead of you (perhaps yourself in the mirror so that you can see what you are doing). Shrug your shoulders up toward your ears. From this position, roll them back and down as far as you can, and hold. That's it. If you are looking in the mirror while doing this, you should see your neck transform from a shy turtle peeking out of its shell to a graceful giraffe. Whenever you aren't sure if you are actually engaging your shoulder blades, do this exercise.

Lower Body

The Language of the Lower Body

A strong lower body means stabilized hip, knee, and ankle joints. It is what carries us, walks us, runs us, lowers us, and stands us up. It dances us. Some of the largest muscles of the body find their home in the lower body. To be able to transport ourselves from any point A to the more desirable point B requires the fervent cooperation of a healthy lower body. This is why we work to strengthen it.

In this book, most of the leg exercises are shown with the Body Bar on the shoulders. Remember that you can always modify any exercise by cradling the bar in front of the body or using the Body Bar for balance.

Wonder Bar

Wondering . . . how to quickly check your alignment when doing squats and lunges? Here are a few fab tricks we find work incredibly well.

If you are not familiar with doing squats or lunges, be sure to include these exercises in your warm-up to remind your body what correct form feels like until you become more comfortable with the movements.

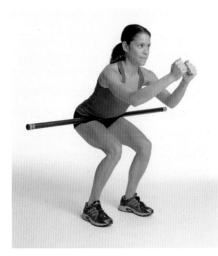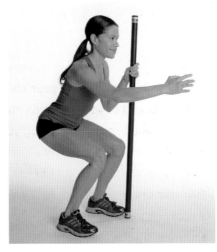

Squat Tricks: (left) Begin in Natural Standing position, with the Body Bar across your hips. When you are down in the squat, the hinge of your hips should hold the bar securely. (right) Hold the Body Bar vertically in front of your big toe. When down in the squat, there should be a small space between the bar and your kneecap.

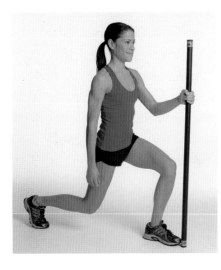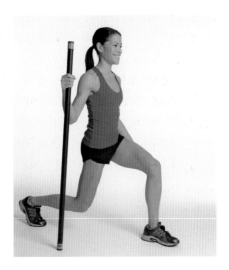

Lunge Tricks: (left) Lower down into a lunge position and hold the Body Bar vertically in front of the big toe of your front leg. There should be a small space between the bar and your kneecap. (right) Hold the Body Bar vertically beside your body with the hand opposite the lunging leg. The top of your head all the way down to your back knee should line up with the bar.

Basic Squat

The Focus: Quadriceps, Hamstrings, Gluteals

The Setup: Begin in Natural Standing Position. Let the Body Bar rest on your trapezius muscle and hold on to the bar with an overhand grip, your hands slightly wider than shoulder width apart.

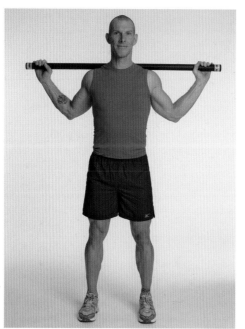 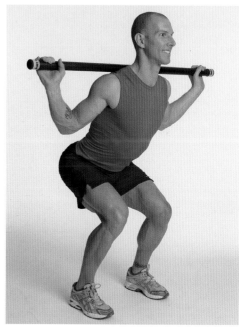

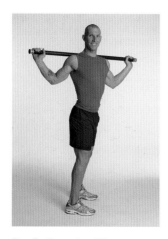

Basic Squat with Rotation

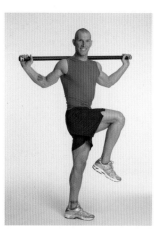

Basic Squat with Rotation and Knee Lift

The Move: Bend your knees and push your hips back as you lower your body as far as you can, creating up to a 90-degree angle at the knees. You should feel your weight over your ankles. Keep your chin lifted off your chest and your focus out in front of you. Imagine pushing the ground away from you as you stand up to starting position.

To Make It Easier: Don't go as deep into the squat.

To Make It Tougher: Add a rotation. Rotate your torso to one side as you stand up to starting position. Keep your hips and knees facing forward throughout this exercise.

To Make It Even Tougher: Lift your knee to hip height or higher. Rotate your torso toward your lifted knee as you come up out of your squat.

Tip: Hinge at the hips as if someone karate chopped you in the waist. At the bottom position of this motion your shoulders should be directly over your knees. Keep your knees aligned with your toes.

Plié Squat

The Focus: Quadriceps, Hamstrings, Gluteals, Adductors

The Setup: Begin with your feet wider than shoulder width apart and with your toes angled out about 45 degrees. Let the Body Bar rest on your trapezius muscle and hold on to the bar with an overhand grip, your hands slightly wider than shoulder width apart.

The Move: Push your hips back slightly as you bend your knees up to 90 degrees and slowly lower into a squat. Keep your chin lifted off your chest and your focus out in front of you. Push into the floor with your heels and squeeze your inner thighs toward each other as you stand up to starting position.

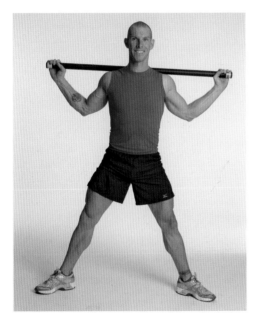 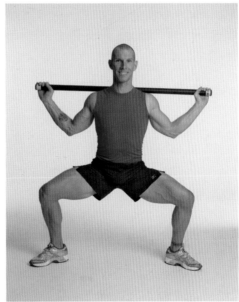

Tips: Keep your toes turned out at a comfortable angle and make sure your toes and knees are aligned throughout the exercise. Keep your weight over your ankles.

Squat with Weight on One Leg

The Focus: Quadriceps, Hamstrings, Gluteals

The Setup: Begin in Natural Standing Position. Let the Body Bar rest on your trapezius muscle and hold on to the bar with an overhand grip, your hands slightly wider than shoulder width apart. Keep your

Doing any type of single-leg squat will help you keep your muscles balanced on both sides since you won't be able to let one side make up for any weaknesses you may have on the other.

elbows directly under your hands. Shift most of your weight to one leg. This will be your working leg. Raise the heel of the opposite leg (your nonworking leg). Keep very little weight on that foot. Use it to help maintain your balance only.

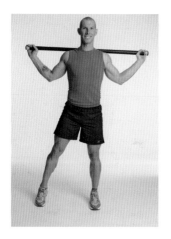

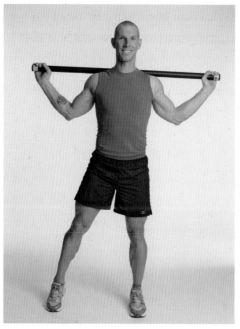

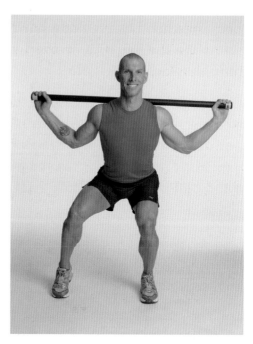

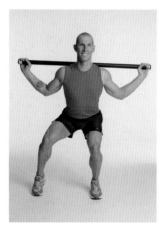

The Move: Bend your knee and push your hips back as you lower your body as far as you can, creating up to a 90-degree angle at the knees. You should feel your weight over the ankle of your working leg. Keep your chin lifted off your chest and your focus out in front of you. Imagine pushing the ground away from you to get back up to starting position.

Tip: To resist putting too much weight on the surface below the nonworking leg, imagine that the surface is fragile.

To Make It Tougher: Try the Frowning Squat version of this exercise: Continuously shift your squat from side to side. As you raise your body out of the squat on one leg, shift your weight to the opposite leg. Repeat the squat on that leg and continue moving fluidly from one leg to the other.

Tips: With the Frowning Squat, imagine drawing a frown in the air with your hips. Keep your knees aligned with your toes.

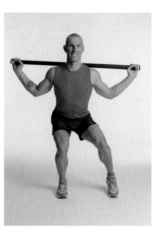

Frowning Squat

Smiley Squat

The Focus: Quadriceps, Hamstrings, Gluteals

The Setup: Begin in Natural Standing Position, but with your feet close together. Let the Body Bar rest on your trapezius muscle and hold on to the bar with an overhand grip, your hands slightly wider than shoulder width apart.

The Move: In one motion, take a wide step sideways, down into a squat, and raise yourself back up to standing position.

Shift your body weight from one foot to the other in a continuous motion. Keep your weight over your ankles, your chin lifted off your chest, and your focus out in front of you.

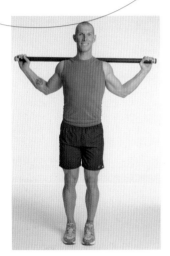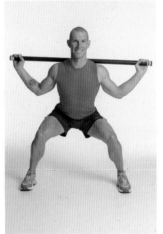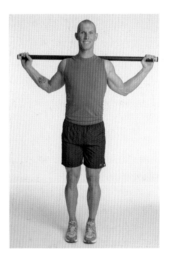

Tip: Imagine drawing a smiley face in the air with your hips.

Uneven Squat to Step-Up

The Focus: Quadriceps, Hamstrings, Gluteals

The Setup: Begin with one foot on the floor and one foot on the platform beside you, your feet between hip and shoulder width apart. Pull your navel in toward your spine, keep your chest lifted, and press your shoulders down and back. Let the Body Bar rest on your trapezius muscle and hold on to the bar with an overhand grip, your hands slightly wider than shoulder width apart.

The Move: Bend your knees and push your hips back as you lower your body as far as you can, creating up to a 90-degree angle at the knees. (At this juncture your working leg is the one on the floor.) You should feel most of your weight over the ankle of that foot. Keep your chin lifted off your chest and your focus out in front of you.

Shift your weight slightly to the elevated leg. Push down into that foot to stand on the platform. (Now your working leg is the one on the platform.) Hold for a moment. Slowly lower yourself to the floor and into the squat position.

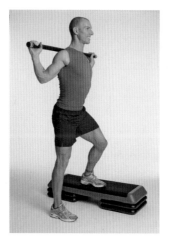 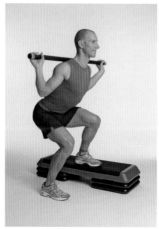 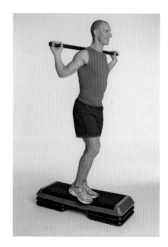

To Make It Tougher: Try using a higher platform or one with an uneven surface such as the Bosu.

Tip: Keep your shoulders, hips, and knees squared off to the front.

Single-Leg Squat

The Focus: Quadriceps, Hamstrings, Gluteals, Hip and Ankle Stability and Balance

The Setup: Begin in Natural Standing Position. Shift most of your weight to one leg. This will be your working leg. Hold the Body Bar like a walking stick in one hand on the side of the nonworking leg, approximately 1 foot in front of you. You will be using the Body Bar for balance in this exercise.

The Move: Push your hips back as you bend the knee of the working leg and lower your body as far as you can, creating up to a 90-degree angle at the knees. Keeping the nonworking leg strong, extend it straight back toward the wall behind you as you are bending. You should feel your weight over the ankle of your working leg. Keep your shoulders down and back, your chin lifted off your chest, and your focus out in front of you. Imagine that you are pushing the floor away with your foot to stand up to starting position. As you lower into the squat, extend the arm holding the bar on a slight angle away from you.

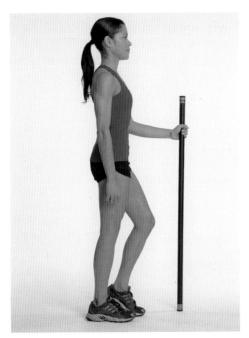 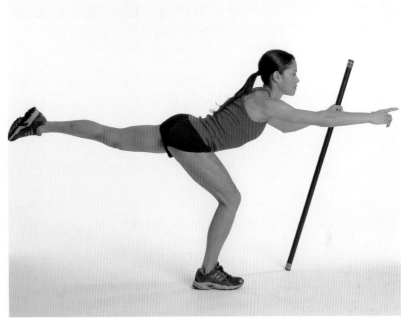

To Make It Tougher: Hold the Body Bar in the hand of the nonworking leg, parallel to the floor. Reach down as if you were going to place the bar on the floor beside you as you squat.

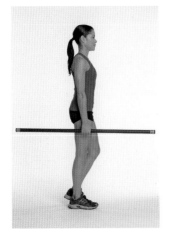 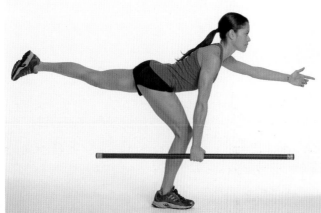

Advanced Single-Leg Squat

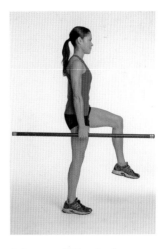

To Make It Even Tougher: Instead of letting the nonworking leg touch the floor in between squats, raise it into a knee lift in front of you.

Tip: Keep your knees aligned with your toes.

Advanced Single-Leg Squat with Knee Lift

Modified Dead Lift

The Focus: Hamstrings, Gluteals, Lower Back

The Setup: Begin in Natural Standing Position. Hold the Body Bar at your hips with an overhand grip, your hands approximately shoulder width apart.

The Move: Bend your knees slightly. Hinge at the hips and slide the bar down your thighs to your knees. Keep your shoulder blades locked into your back, your chin lifted off your chest, and your focus forward. You should feel most of your weight over your ankles. Imagine that you are pushing the floor away with your feet as you push your hips forward to stand up to starting position.

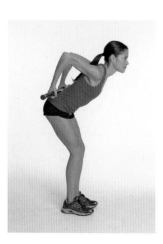

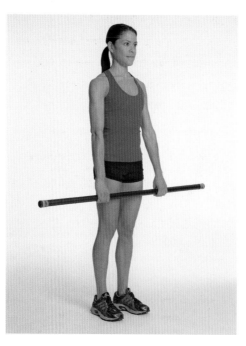

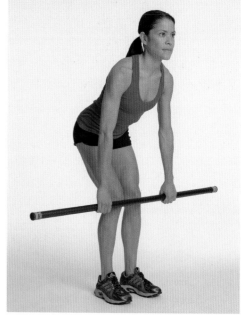

Easier Modified Dead Lift

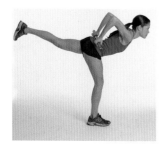

Modified Single-Leg Dead Lift

To Make It Easier: Try holding the Body Bar behind you. Rest it on the base of your lower back. Keep your hands wide, and hold the bar with an underhand grip.

To Make It Tougher: Try this on one leg. As you hinge at the hips, reach the nonworking leg straight back toward the wall behind you. Your upper body and your nonworking leg will be as close to parallel to the floor as possible. Push into the floor to stand up to starting position. This exercise will help develop ankle and hip stability as well as overall balance.

Tips: The angle of your knee should remain fixed throughout this exercise. If you need help keeping your balance when doing this exercise on one leg, use the bar in a walking-stick style.

Dead Lift

The Focus: Hamstrings, Gluteals, Lower Back

The Setup: Begin in Natural Standing Position. Hold the Body Bar at your hips with an overhand grip, your hands wider than shoulder width apart.

The Move: Bend your knees, push your hips back, and slide the bar down your thighs as if you wanted to put the bar on the floor. You should be in a squat position with the bar slightly lower than knee height. Keep your shoulder blades locked into your back, your chin lifted off your chest, and your focus forward. You should feel most of your weight over your ankles. Drive your feet into the floor as you push your hips forward to stand up to starting position.

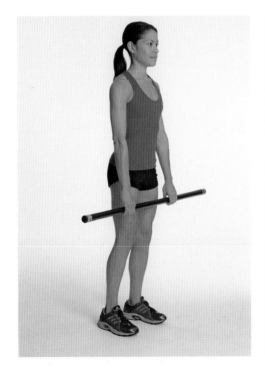 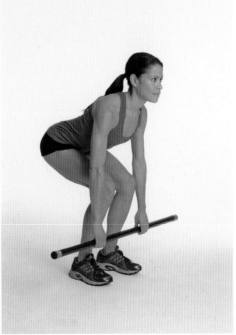

Tips: Pay extra attention to keeping your back flat throughout the motion of the dead lift. Imagine reaching your tailbone and your shoulder blades toward each other.

Front Step-Up

The Focus: Quadriceps, Hamstrings, Gluteals

The Setup: Begin with one foot on the floor and one foot on the platform in front of you. Let the Body Bar rest on your trapezius muscle and hold on to the bar with an overhand grip, your hands wider than shoulder width apart.

The Move: Push into the foot on the platform to step up. Hold for a moment and slowly lower to starting position.

For a Change: You can also do the same exercise with the platform on one side of you.

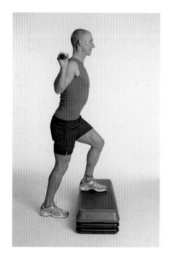 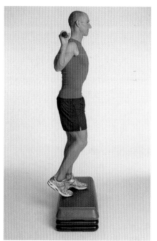 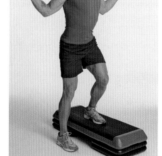 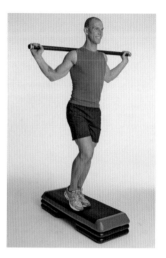

Front Step-Up   **Side Step-Up**

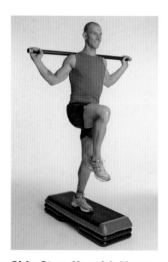

To Make It Tougher: Lift the knee of the nonworking leg up to hip height as you step up to the platform. Also, try using a higher platform.

Tip: Step the back foot to the floor lightly, transferring very little body weight to that foot.

Side Step-Up with Knee Lift

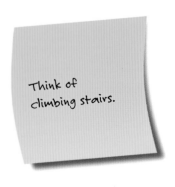

Think of climbing stairs.

Basic Lunge

The Focus: Quadriceps, Hamstrings, Gluteals

The Setup: Begin in Natural Standing Position. Let the Body Bar rest on your trapezius muscle and hold on to the bar with an overhand grip, your hands slightly wider than shoulder width apart. Take a large step forward straight ahead. Your weight should be evenly distributed between both feet.

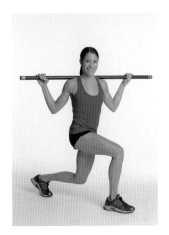

Basic Lunge with Rotation

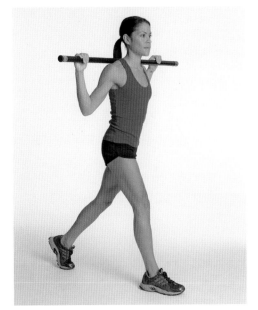
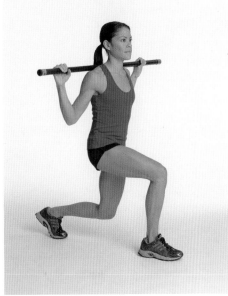

The Move: Bend both knees and lower your hips straight to the floor. Most of your weight should now be over the ankle of your front leg, and your back heel will be off the floor. Your front knee should be bent up to 90 degrees. Imagine that you are pushing the floor away with your feet to return to starting position.

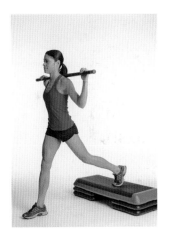

To Make It Tougher: Rotate your torso toward the front leg as you lower into the lunge.

To Make It Even Tougher: Try a lunge with your back leg up on a low platform.

In essence, a lunge is a squat with a split stance. When doing any type of lunge, keep your knees aligned with your toes. Be extra careful that your knee does not extend beyond your toes. If in doubt of your form, refer back to the squat and lunge alignment tricks in the Wonder Bar earlier in this chapter.

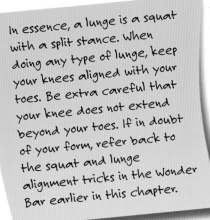

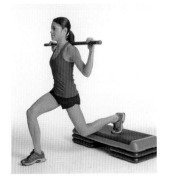

Lunge with Rear Leg Elevation

Forward Lunge

The Focus: Quadriceps, Hamstrings, Gluteals

The Setup: Begin in Natural Standing Position. Let the Body Bar rest on your trapezius muscle and hold on to the bar with an overhand grip, your hands slightly wider than shoulder width apart.

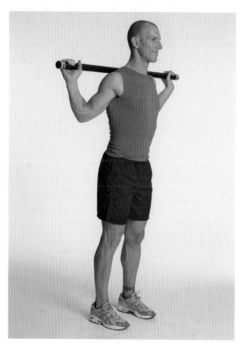 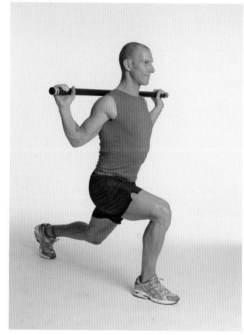

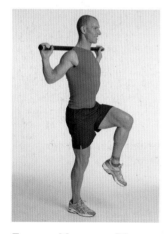

Forward Lunge with Rotation

The Move: Take a large step forward straight ahead, bend both knees, and lower your hips straight to the floor. Most of your weight will be over the ankle of your front leg, and your back heel will be off the floor. Your front knee should be bent up to 90 degrees. Push off the floor with enough force to return your body to starting position.

To Make It Tougher: Rotate your torso approximately 45 degrees toward the front leg as you step.

Reverse Lunge

The Focus: Quadriceps, Hamstrings, Gluteals.

By shifting your weight backward in the reverse lunge, you add an aspect of coordination to the exercise.

The Setup: Begin in Natural Standing Position. Let the Body Bar rest on your trapezius muscle and hold on to the bar with an overhand grip, your hands slightly wider than shoulder width apart.

The Move: Take a step straight backward, keeping your body weight over the ankle of your front leg. Bend both knees and lower your hips straight to the floor. Most of your weight will be over the ankle of your front leg, and your back heel will be off the floor. Your front knee should be bent up to 90 degrees. Push down into the ground with your front foot to stand up to starting position.

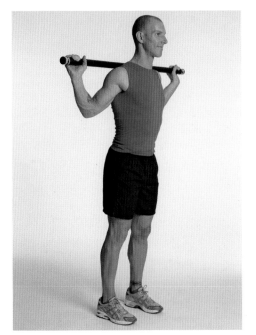
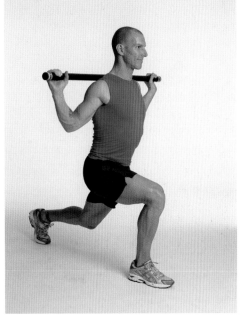
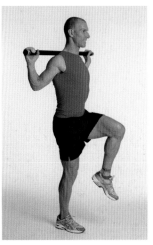

Reverse Lunge with Knee Lift

To Make It Tougher: Try lifting your knee to hip height as you stand.

Reverse Lunge from Platform

The Focus: Quadriceps, Hamstrings, Gluteals

The Setup: Begin in Natural Standing Position on a platform. Let the Body Bar rest on your trapezius muscle and hold on to the bar with an overhand grip, your hands slightly wider than shoulder width apart.

The Move: Take a step straight backward off the platform, keeping your body weight over the ankle of your front leg. Bend both knees and lower your hips straight to the floor. Most of your weight will be over the ankle of your front leg, and your back heel will be off the

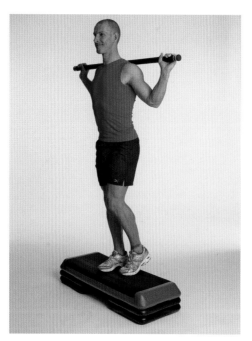 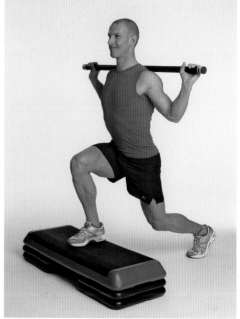

floor. Your front knee should be bent up to 90 degrees. Push down into the ground with your front foot to stand up to starting position on the platform.

To Make It Tougher: Try lifting your knee to hip height as you stand back up on the platform.

Tip: Don't push off your back leg.

Side Lunge

The Focus: Quadriceps, Hamstrings, Gluteals

The Setup: Begin in Natural Standing Position. Let the Body Bar rest on your trapezius muscle and hold on to the bar with an overhand grip, your hands slightly wider than shoulder width apart.

The Move: Take a large step (approximately 2 to 3 feet) out to one side. Push your hips back and bend your knee up to 90 degrees. Keep both feet facing forward and your nonlunging leg straight. Most of your weight will be over the ankle of your lunging leg. Keep your shoulder blades locked into your back, your chin lifted off your chest, and your focus forward. Push off the floor with enough force to return your body to starting position.

To Make It Easier: Try using the bar for balance. Hold the Body Bar

This exercise will give your glutes a serious burn.

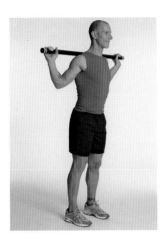 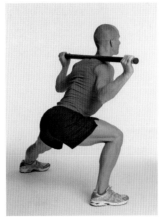 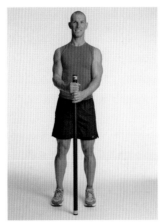 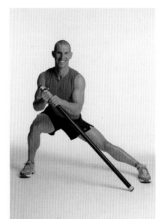

Easier Side Lunge

vertically in front of you. As you lunge, push the bar into the ground for added stability.

Tip: Keep the lunging knee aligned with your toes.

Curtsy Lunge

The Focus: Quadriceps, Hamstrings, Gluteals

The Setup: Begin in Natural Standing Position. Let the Body Bar rest on your trapezius muscle and hold on to the bar with an overhand grip, your hands slightly wider than shoulder width apart.

The Move: Shift your weight to one side. Step backward in a diagonal line behind your standing leg, bend both knees, and lower your hips

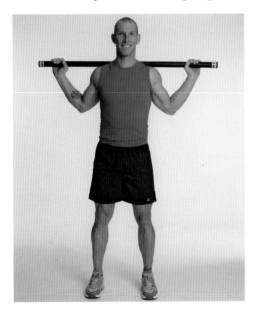 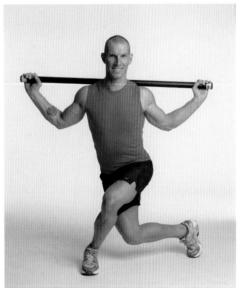

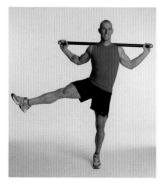

Curtsy Lunge with Kick

directly to the floor until your front knee is bent up to 90 degrees. Most of your weight will be over the ankle of your front foot, and your back heel will be off the floor. Push down into the ground with your front foot to stand up to starting position. Don't forget to keep your chest lifted and your gaze forward.

To Make It Tougher: Don't rest your back foot on the floor when you stand up to starting position. Lift it out to the side.

Tip: When you are down in the Curtsy Lunge, your back knee should be directly behind the lower part of your front leg.

Standing Forward Leg Lift

The Focus: Hip Flexors, Abdominal Muscles as Spinal Stabilizers

The Setup: Begin in Natural Standing Position. Bring one leg forward and point your toe. Turn your heel in toward your center line (the center of your body). Rest the bottom of the Body Bar in the arch of your foot. Support that position by holding the top of the bar with your hand.

The Move: Slowly and with control, lift your leg as high as you can. Hold for a moment and slowly lower to starting position.

Tips: Stand tall and keep both legs straight, but don't lock your knees. Be careful not to lean backward. Give extra focus to keeping your abs engaged.

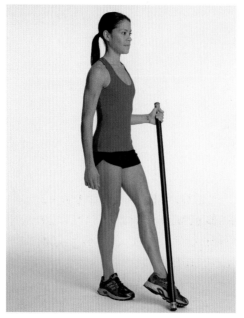
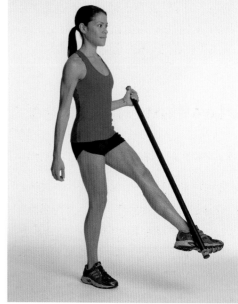

Standing Side Leg Lift

The Focus: Abductors

The Setup: Begin in Natural Standing Position. Rest the bottom of the Body Bar on the outside of one foot near the ankle. Support it in that position by holding the top of the bar with your hand.

The Move: Slowly and with control lift your leg out to the side as high as you can. Hold for a moment and slowly lower to starting position.

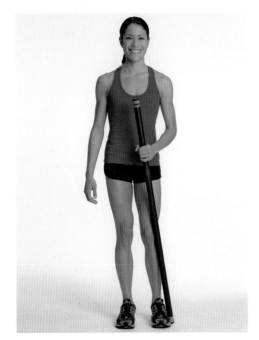 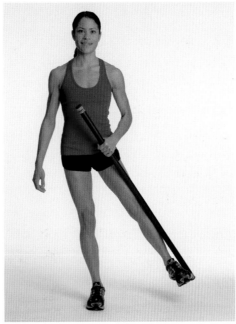

Tips: Keep both legs straight, but don't lock your knees. The Leaning Tower of Pisa is not the thing to mimic while doing this exercise. There should be no leaning to the side as you lift your leg. Keep your body upright and your hips squared and level throughout this exercise.

Standing Rear Leg Lift

The Focus: Gluteals, Hamstrings

The Setup: Begin in Natural Standing Position. Point your toe and bring one leg straight out behind you. Rest the bottom of the Body Bar above the heel of your back leg. Support the bar in that position by holding the top of the bar with your hand.

To make any of the standing leg lift exercises tougher, don't let your foot rest on the floor at the bottom of the rep.

The Move: Slowly and with control lift your back leg behind you as high as you can. Hold for a moment and slowly lower to starting position.

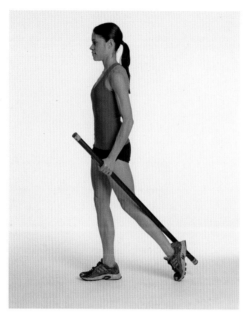 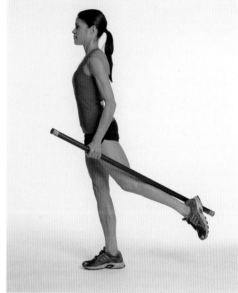

Tips: Don't lean forward. Stand tall. Remember to keep your chest lifted throughout this exercise. Use your glutes and hamstrings to lift your leg. Keep your pelvis in a neutral position.

Side-Lying Leg Lift

The Focus: Abductors

The Setup: Lie on one side with your head resting on your arm. Keep your head, shoulders, and hips in one line, with your navel pulled in toward the spine. Rest the bottom of the Body Bar on the top foot and support it in that position with your free hand.

The Move: Slowly and with control, lift your top leg up to a 45-degree angle. Hold for a moment and slowly lower to starting position.

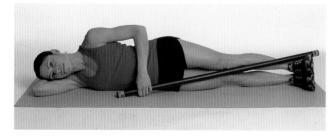 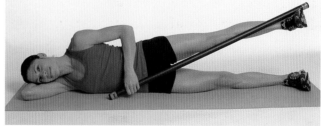

Tip: The farther away you push the bar out over your foot, the heavier it is and the more difficult this exercise.

Side-Lying Inner Thigh Lift

The Focus: Adductors

The Setup: Lie on one side with your head resting on your arm. Keep your head, shoulders, and hips in one line, with your navel pulled in toward your spine. Rest one end of the Body Bar on the arch of your bottom foot. Rest the other end on the floor and support it in that position with your free hand. Bend the knee of the top leg. Rotate that leg open and place your foot flat on the floor behind your front leg.

The Move: Slowly and with control, lift your lower leg. Keep your leg fully extended throughout the movement. Hold for a moment and slowly lower back to starting position.

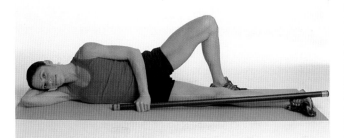 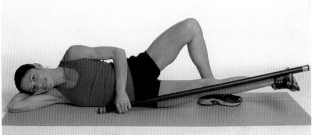

Tip: The farther away you push the bar out over your foot, the more of its weight your leg will be supporting and the more difficult this exercise will be.

Bridge

The Focus: Hamstrings, Gluteals, Lower Back, Abdominal Muscles

The Setup: Lie on your back with both feet resting on a platform in front of you. Your knees should be bent about 90 degrees. Balance the Body Bar across your hips, stabilizing it with your hands.

The Move: Drive your feet into the platform and push your hips up until your body forms a straight line from knees to shoulders. Keep your shoulders on the floor. Hold for a moment and lower to starting position.

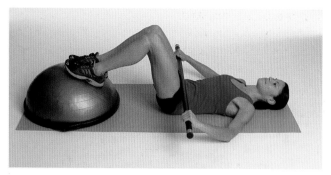 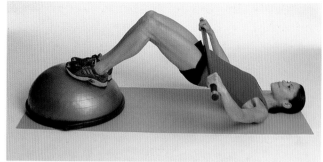

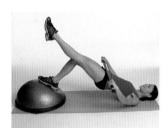

Bridge with Leg Extension

To Make It Tougher: Lift one foot off the platform and straighten your leg. Keep your knees in line with each other. Keep the leg lifted throughout the exercise. You can also try the static version of this exercise: Hold your hips and leg in the lifted position for 10 to 60 seconds. Don't forget to work both sides evenly.

Tip: Keep your hips aligned throughout this exercise.

Calf Raise

The Focus: Calves

The Setup: Begin in Natural Standing Position. Position the bar vertically on the floor in front of you, holding the top of it with one hand.

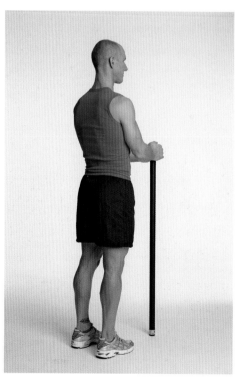 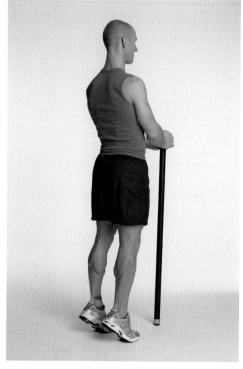

The Move: Lift your heels off the floor as far as you can until you are on the balls of your feet. Keep your legs straight. Hold at the peak of the contraction for a moment, and slowly and with control lower your heels to the floor.

To Make It Tougher: Try this exercise with the bar across your shoulders, or keep the bar in front of you but balance on one leg at a time.

Bent-Knee Calf Raise

The Focus: Calves. This version of the calf raise will put more emphasis on the deeper calf muscle. It is also an isometric contraction for the hips and legs.

The Setup: Begin in a squat position. Hold the bar out in front of you with fully extended arms. Keep your back as upright as possible with your chin lifted off your chest.

The Move: Hold the squat position and lift your heels off the floor as far as you can until you are on the balls of your feet. Hold at the peak of the contraction for a moment. Slowly and with control lower your heels to the floor.

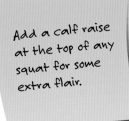

Add a calf raise at the top of any squat for some extra flair.

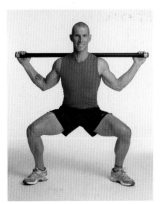

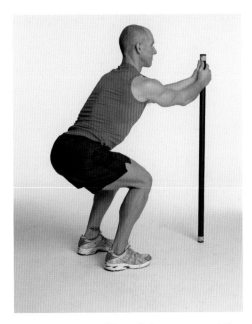

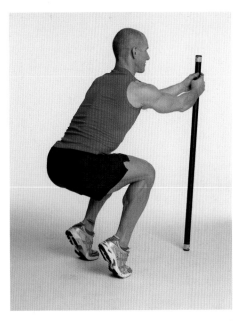

For a Change: Try this move with your legs wide and your feet angled out to the sides (holding at the bottom of a plié squat).

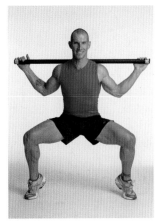

Plié Squat with Calf Raise

Speed Skater

The Focus: Quadriceps, Hamstrings, Gluteals

The Setup: Begin in Natural Standing Position. Let the Body Bar rest on your lower back just above your hips, and hold the bar near the ends with a wide underhand grip. Bend your knees and push your hips back to a semisquat position.

The Move: Push off one foot, leaping sideways in a gliding motion to the other foot. Be sure to stay in the squat position throughout the entire motion.

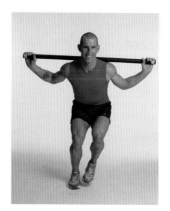 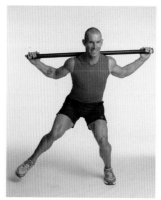 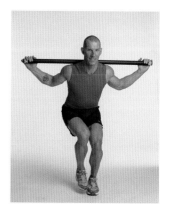

To Make It Easier: Try this move without the bar. It is still very effective.

To Make It Tougher: Stay in the deepest squat possible, accelerate the speed of the movement, and extend the width of your leap.

Tips: Keep your back flat throughout this movement. Imagine that you are on in-line skates.

Crab Walk

The Focus: Quadriceps, Hamstrings, Gluteals

The Setup: Begin in a squat position with your feet wider than shoulder width apart. Let the Body Bar rest on your trapezius muscle and hold on to the bar with an overhand grip, your hands slightly wider than shoulder width apart.

The Move: Take two to four big shuffle steps to one direction, and then back to the starting point.

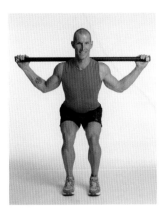 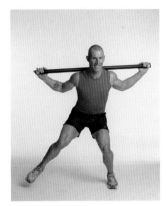 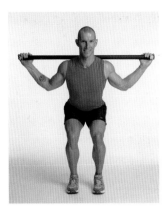

To Make It Tougher: Stay in the deepest squat possible, accelerate the speed of the movement, and extend the width of your step.

Tips: Keep your shoulder blades down and back, your chin lifted off your chest, and your focus forward throughout this move.

The Upper Body

The upper body is our facilitator. It is what allows us the immediate control of permitting that which attracts us to come closest, and it is what we use to protect ourselves. We extend our arms to draw things to us, and push away that which we reject. It is all the parts that reach and hold, push and pull, lift and carry. In its strength, we bring ease to its functions.

Back

Narrow-Grip Bent-Over Row

The Focus: Latissimus Dorsi, Posterior Deltoids, Biceps

The Setup: Begin in Natural Standing Position. Hold the Body Bar with a narrow, underhand grip. Hinge at your hips until your thighs and torso form a 90-degree angle. Keep your back as flat as possible by engaging your shoulder blades into your back. It should feel like you are puffing your chest out. Let the bar hang straight down to the floor.

Rowing exercises will strengthen some of the muscles vital in supporting good posture. Doing a combination of different types of rows will increase the overall strength of your back.

The Move: Pull the bar up to just below your navel, keeping your elbows tucked in and close to the sides of your body throughout the exercise. Hold for a moment and slowly lower to starting position.

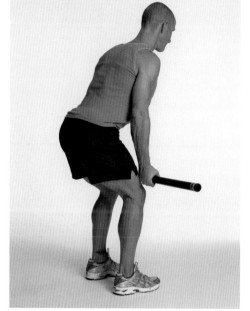 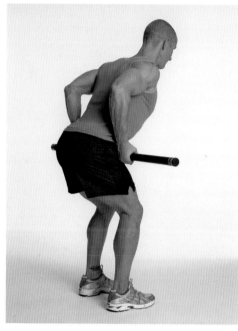

To Make It Tougher: You can do this exercise unilaterally (one arm at a time). Hold the middle of the Body Bar at your side with an overhand grip. Step the leg on the same side back approximately 3 steps. Let the bar hang straight down to the floor. Pull your hand back to your hip, keeping your elbow tucked in and close to the side of your body throughout the exercise. Hold for a moment and slowly lower to starting position.

Tips: To help maintain a flat back, imagine a line streaming out of the top of your head in one direction, and out through the base of your spine in the other. For extra support for your lower back when doing the single-arm version, rest the hand of your nonworking arm on your thigh. Squeeze your shoulder blades together tightly. Be careful not to shrug your shoulders.

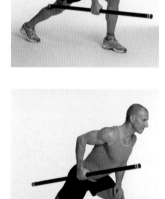

Single-Arm Narrow-Grip Bent-Over Row

Wide-Grip Bent-Over Row

The Focus: Posterior Deltoids, Upper Back, Elbow Flexors

The Setup: Begin in Natural Standing Position. Hold the Body Bar wider than shoulder width apart with an overhand grip. Hinge forward at the hips until your thighs and torso form a 90-degree angle. Keep your back as flat as possible by engaging your shoulder blades into your back. It should feel like you are puffing your chest out. Let the bar hang straight down to the floor.

The Move: Using the muscles of your back, drive your elbows out and up in a sweeping motion. Pull the bar up to the top of your abs. Hold for a moment and slowly lower to starting position.

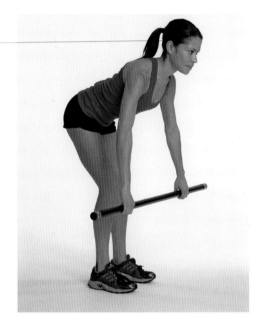 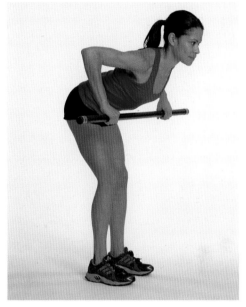

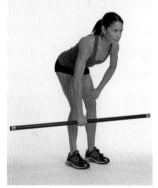

To Make It Tougher: You can do this exercise unilaterally. Hold the middle of the Body Bar with an overhand grip at your side. Step the leg on the same side back approximately 3 steps. Let the bar hang straight down to the floor. Using the muscles of the back, drive your elbow out and up in a sweeping motion. Pull the bar up to the top of your abs. Hold for a moment and slowly lower to starting position.

Tips: At the top of the movement, your elbows should be directly out to your sides at shoulder height. To help maintain a flat back, imagine a line streaming out of the top of your head in one direction, and out through the base of your spine in the other. As you pull the bar, squeeze your shoulder blades together as if you were trying to hold a pencil between them. For extra support for your lower back when doing the unilateral version, rest the hand of your nonworking arm on your thigh.

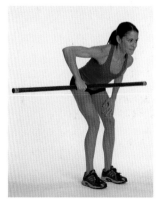

Single-Arm Wide-Grip Bent-Over Row

Pullover

The Focus: Latissimus Dorsi, Posterior Deltoids, Upper Back, Pectorals, Triceps

The Setup: Lie on your back on a platform with both feet resting squarely on the floor in front of you. Pull your navel in toward your spine. Hold the Body Bar with an overhand grip above your chest, your hands shoulder width apart. Keep your elbows slightly bent.

The Move: Slowly lower the Body Bar in an arc over your head toward the floor behind you until you feel a comfortable stretch at your sides and through your abs. Hold for a moment and slowly bring the bar back in the same arc to the starting position.

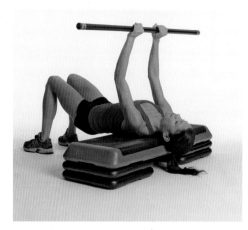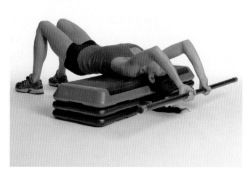

To Make It Tougher: Try this exercise unilaterally. Be sure to have mastered the bilateral movement and feel completely comfortable moving on. The unilateral version will be a much bigger challenge for your shoulder stabilizers. Hold the middle of the Body Bar in one hand with an overhand grip.

Tips: The bend in your elbows should not change throughout this exercise. Give your abs extra attention to avoid hyperextension of the lower back. Keep your shoulder blades firmly locked into your back.

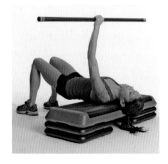

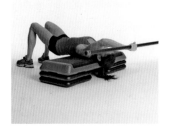

Single-Arm Pullover

Chest

Push-Up

The Focus: Pectorals, Anterior Deltoids, Triceps, Core Stability

The Setup: Kneel behind your platform with the Body Bar lying across it. Hold the Body Bar with an overhand grip, your hands wider than shoulder width apart. Keep your wrists straight and strong. Contract your navel in toward your spine. Straighten your legs so that your weight is supported on your toes and your hands and your body is in a straight line from your head to your toes.

The Move: Bend your elbows to a 90-degree angle or farther, lowering the middle of your chest over the Body Bar. Push up to starting position.

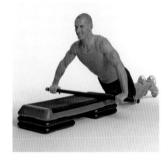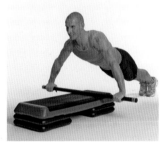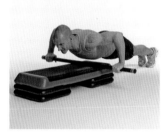

To Make It Tougher: Try this with your hands closer together, approximately shoulder width apart. As you lower the middle of your chest toward the bar, keep your elbows close to the sides of your body. This will be a bigger challenge for your triceps than doing a push-up with your hands positioned wide apart.

If you are unable to do a full push-up, here is a good way to work up to it. First, try a push-up from your knees instead of your toes.

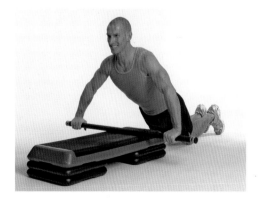

Wonder Bar

Wondering . . . how to correctly pronounce the name of this push-up? The correct pronunciation is "e-sen-trick," and not "eccentric," as in unusual. It is a very practical way to build up to a full push-up, but it does seem like a rather odd, multiplex way of doing a push-up.

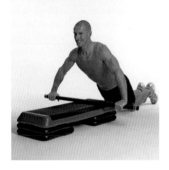

Once you have mastered this and can do 15 to 20 reps from your knees, try this: Begin, once again, on your knees. Straighten your legs and lower your chest to the bar; then drop your knees to the floor and push up to starting position.

Tip: Imagine pushing the bar into the platform.

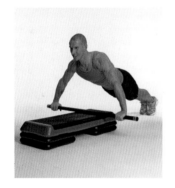 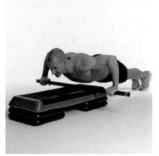 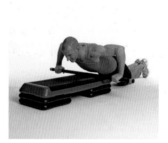 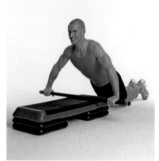

Eccentric Push-Up

Chest Press

The Focus: Pectorals, Anterior Deltoids, Triceps

The Setup: Lie on your back on a platform with both feet resting squarely on the floor in front of you. Pull your navel in toward your spine. Hold the Body Bar with an overhand grip above your chest, your hands slightly wider than shoulder width apart. Keep your arms fully extended but your elbows unlocked.

The Move: Slowly lower the Body Bar to the middle of your chest. Press the bar up to starting position.

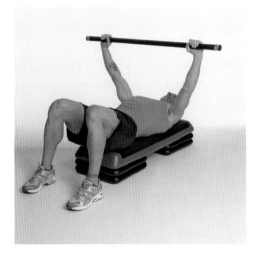
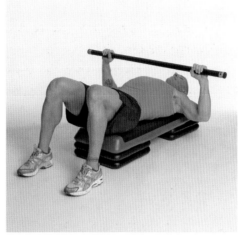

To Make It Tougher: Try this exercise unilaterally. Be sure to have mastered the bilateral movement and feel completely comfortable moving on. The unilateral version will be a much bigger challenge for your shoulder stabilizers. Hold the middle of the Body Bar in one hand with an overhand grip. Your arm should be directly over your shoulder at the top of this exercise. As you lower the Body Bar to the middle of your chest, your elbow should create an arc directly out to the side of the shoulder. Slowly press the bar up to starting position.

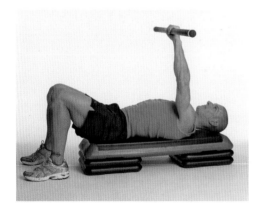
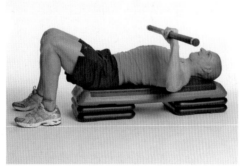

Single-Arm Chest Press

Tips: As you press the bar up to starting position, imagine pushing your body down into the bench. Keep your wrists straight and strong.

Narrow-Grip Chest Press

The Focus: Pectorals, Triceps. This exercise puts more emphasis on the inner part of your chest.

The Setup: Lie on your back on a platform with both feet resting squarely on the floor in front of you. Pull your navel in toward your spine. Hold the Body Bar above your chest with an overhand grip, your hands shoulder width apart or slightly closer together. Keep your arms fully extended and your elbows unlocked.

The Move: Slowly lower the Body Bar to just below the middle of your chest. Keep your elbows close to your sides. Slowly press the bar up to starting position.

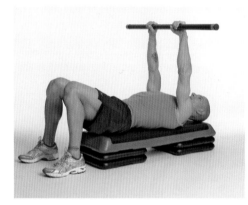 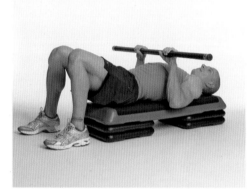

To Make It Tougher: Try this exercise unilaterally. Be sure to have mastered the bilateral movement and feel completely comfortable moving on. The unilateral version will be a much bigger challenge for your shoulder stabilizers. Hold the middle of the Body Bar in one hand with an overhand grip. Your arm should be directly over your shoulder at the top of the exercise.

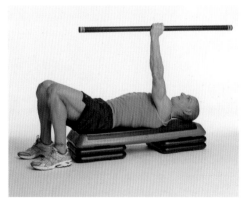 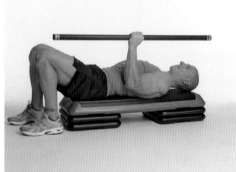

Single-Arm Narrow-Grip Chest Press

Single-Arm Chest Fly

The Focus: Pectorals (specifically the inner part), Anterior Deltoids

The Setup: Lie on your back on a platform with both feet resting squarely on the floor in front of you. Pull your navel in toward your spine. Hold the middle of the Body Bar in one hand, parallel to your body and above your shoulder. Keep your arm slightly bent.

The Move: Lower the Body Bar in an arc directly out to the side of your body until you feel a comfortable stretch in your pectoral muscles. Slowly bring the bar up in the same arc to starting position.

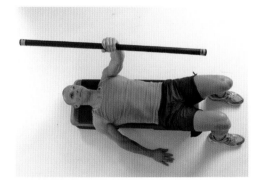 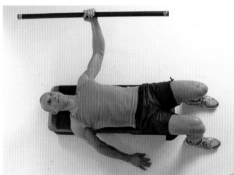

For a Change: If you have access to two bars, you can work both sides at the same time.

Tips: The bend in your elbow should not change throughout this exercise. When you use one bar for this exercise, imagine that you are painting half a rainbow with your arm. When you use two bars, imagine you are hugging a big tree.

Shoulders

Shoulder Press

The Focus: Anterior Deltoids, Trapezius, Triceps

The Setup: Begin in Natural Standing Position. Hold the Body Bar at shoulder height with an overhand grip, your hands slightly wider than shoulder width apart.

All the chest exercises performed lying on a platform can also be done lying directly on the floor or on a mat, if that is all you have to work with. The exercises will be effective, but not as effective, because you will not be getting as full a range of motion. If you are doing these exercises on a Bosu, you will need to lift your hips so that your body is in a straight line from the top of your head to your knees, like a table or a bridge.

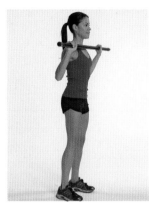

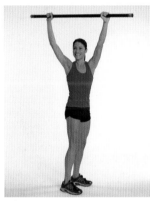

Shoulder Press Rotation

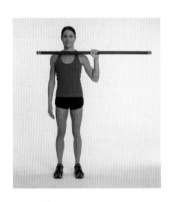

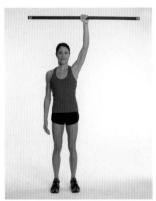

Single-Arm Shoulder Press

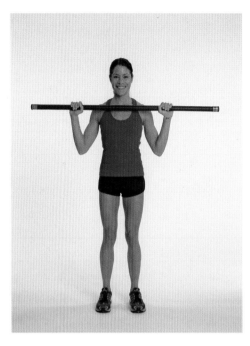

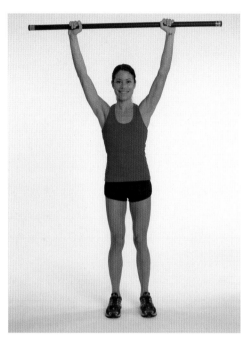

The Move: Push the bar toward the ceiling until your arms are fully extended but not locked. Hold for a moment and slowly lower to starting position.

To Make It Tougher: Rotate your torso about 45 degrees as you press. Work to keep your hips facing forward.

You can also make this move tougher by doing this exercise unilaterally, which will put more emphasis on shoulder stabilization. Hold the middle of the Body Bar in one hand with an overhand grip at shoulder height, with your elbow out to the side. Push the bar in an arc toward the ceiling until your arm is fully extended but not locked. Hold for a moment and slowly lower in the same arc to starting position.

Tips: In any type of shoulder press, as you push the bar up imagine pushing your shoulder blades down your back, creating a long feeling in the neck. When doing this exercise with one arm, concentrate on keeping the movement slow, smooth, and controlled.

Pendulum

The Focus: Medial Deltoids

The Setup: Begin in Natural Standing Position. Hold the Body Bar with an extra-wide relaxed overhand grip in front of your hips. Keep your elbows slightly bent and your wrists straight and strong.

The Move: Lift the bar in a sweeping arc out to the side and up to shoulder height. Hold for a moment and slowly lower in the same arc to starting position.

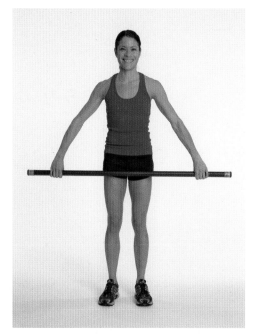 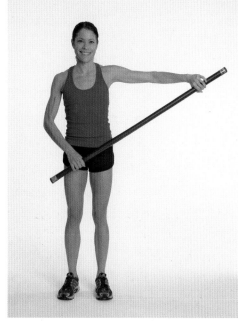

Tips: Keep your elbows directly in line with your shoulders throughout this exercise. Imagine your elbows being pulled up to the ceiling by a string. As you lift the bar out to the side, loosen your grip slightly so that your wrists stay in a neutral position. At that point you should be holding the bar primarily with your thumb and index finger. Let the working arm carry most of the weight. If necessary, use the nonworking arm to support the motion.

Lateral Raise

The Focus: Medial Deltoids

The Setup: Begin in Natural Standing Position. Hold the middle of the Body Bar with an overhand grip at your side, slightly forward of your shoulder. Keep your elbows slightly bent and your wrists straight and strong.

The Move: Lift the bar in a sweeping arc out to the side and up to shoulder height. Hold for a moment and slowly lower in the same arc to starting position.

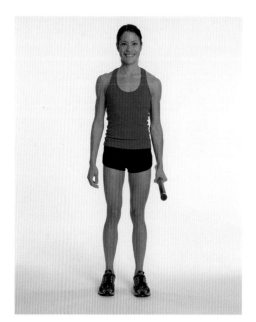 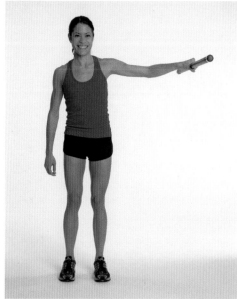

Tips: You will probably need to use a lighter bar to do this exercise. Keep your elbow directly in line with your shoulder throughout this exercise. Imagine your elbows being pulled up to the ceiling by a string. This exercise is a good alternative to the Pendulum.

Rear Shoulder Extension

The Focus: Posterior Deltoids

The Setup: Begin in Natural Standing Position. Hold the Body Bar behind your back with an overhand grip. Lock your shoulder blades into your back; keep your chin lifted off your chest and your focus forward.

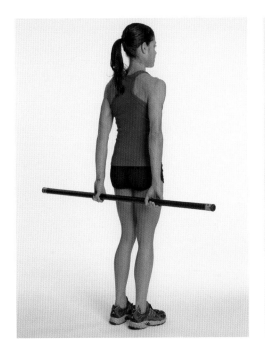
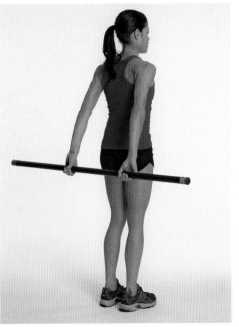
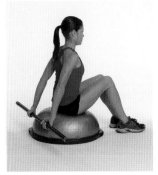
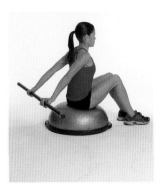

The Move: Press the bar away from your body in an upward arc approximately 3 to 6 inches. Keep your elbows extended and unlocked. Hold for a moment and slowly return to starting position.

To Make It Easier: Try this exercise seated.

Tips: Keep your torso tall throughout the movement. Resist rocking forward as you press the bar away.

Seated Rear Shoulder Extension

Single-Arm Rear Deltoid Fly

The Focus: Posterior Deltoids

The Setup: Begin in Natural Standing Position. Hold the middle of the Body Bar with an overhand grip at your side. Hinge at the hips up to a 90-degree angle. Keep your elbows slightly bent and your back as flat as possible. It should feel like you are puffing your chest out. Let the bar hang straight down to the floor.

The Move: Lift the bar in a sweeping arc out to the side up to shoulder height. Hold for a moment and slowly lower in the same arc to starting position.

To Make It Easier: Rest one end of the bar on the floor behind you. You can also try this exercise lying facedown on a high platform or seated, hinged at the hips with your chest leaning over your thighs. If

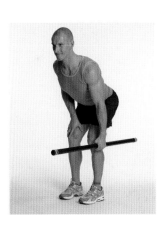
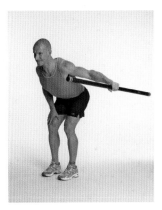

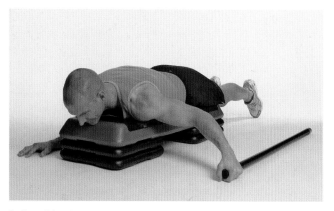 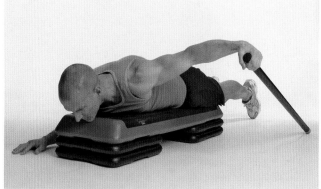

Lying Single-Arm Rear Deltoid Fly

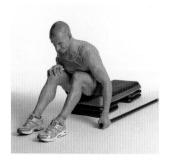

you have access to two bars, you can work both sides at the same time.

Tips: You will probably need to use a lighter bar for this exercise. For more support for your lower back, rest the hand of your nonworking arm on your thigh. To help maintain a flat back, imagine a line streaming out of the top of your head in one direction and out through the base of your spine in the other. Keep your wrists straight and strong.

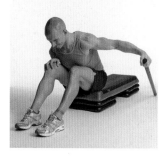

Seated Single-Arm Rear Deltoid Fly

Front Raise

The Focus: Anterior Deltoids

The Setup: Begin in Natural Standing Position. Hold the Body Bar at your hips with an overhand grip, your hands shoulder width apart. Keep your elbows slightly bent.

The Move: Lock your shoulder blades into your back. Lift the bar in a sweeping arc out in front of your body up to shoulder height. Hold for a moment and slowly lower back in the same arc to starting position.

Tips: Pay extra attention to locking your shoulder blades into your back. With this exercise, there is a strong tendency toward shrugging the shoulders. If you are unable to do this exercise without your shoulders creeping up to your ears, choose a lighter bar.

To Make It Tougher: Try doing this exercise unilaterally. Hold the bar at your side with an overhand grip and keep your elbows slightly bent. Lift the bar in a sweeping arc out in front of your body, slightly

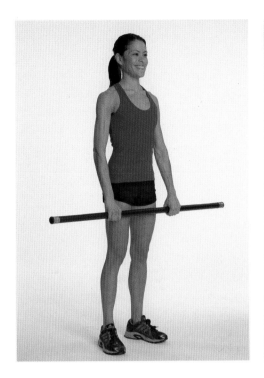

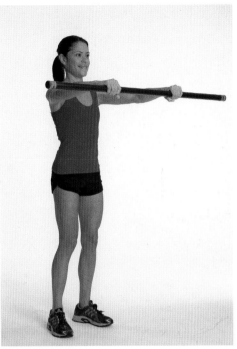

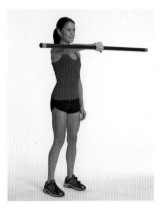

Single Arm Front Raise

wider than your shoulder. Hold for a moment and slowly lower in the same arc to starting position.

Tips: As you lift the weight in front of your body, pay attention to your core. Be sure to stand upright and keep your upper torso still. Avoid rocking backward to lift the bar.

Reverse-Grip Front Raise

The Focus: Anterior Deltoids, Biceps

The Setup: Begin in Natural Standing Position. Hold the Body Bar just below your navel with an underhand grip, your hands shoulder width apart. Keep your elbows bent almost 90 degrees.

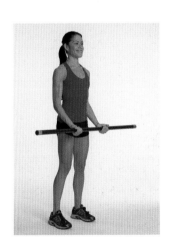

The Move: Lock your shoulder blades into your back. Lift the bar in a sweeping arc out in front of your body until the bar is at approximately eye level. Hold for a moment and slowly lower in the same arc to starting position.

Tips: Focus extra attention on your core, especially as you lift the weight in front of your body. Be sure to stand upright and keep your upper torso still. Avoid rocking backward to lift the bar. At the top of the movement, your forearms will be almost perpendicular to the floor.

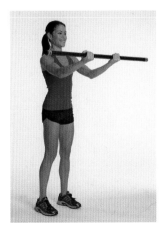

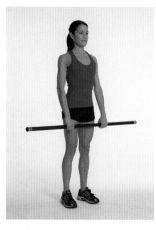

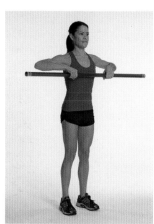

Modified Upright Row

The Focus: Anterior Deltoids, Medial Deltoids, Trapezius

The Setup: Begin in Natural Standing Position. Hold the Body Bar at your hips with an overhand grip, your hands shoulder width apart.

The Move: Lock your shoulder blades into your back. Lift the bar, keeping it close to your body until your elbows are at shoulder height. Hold for a moment and slowly lower to starting position.

Tips: As you pull the bar up, imagine sliding your shoulder blades down and into your back, creating a long feeling in your neck. Your elbows should always be above the bar.

Wave

The Focus: Anterior Deltoids, Biceps

The Setup: Begin in Natural Standing Position. Hold the Body Bar at your hips with an overhand grip, your hands shoulder width apart.

The Move: Lock your shoulder blades into your back. Lift the bar, keeping it close to your body until your elbows are at shoulder height. Push the bar out in front of you until your arms are fully extended, and in a smooth, sweeping arc slowly lower the bar to starting position.

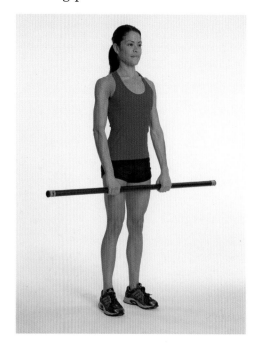

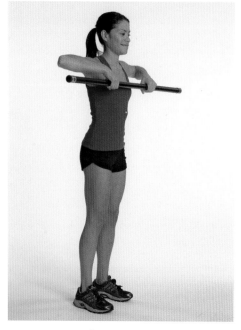

(continued on next page)

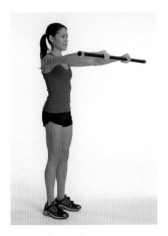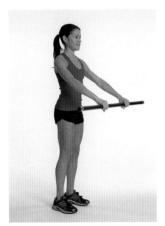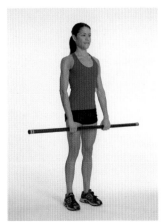

Wave (cont.)

Tip: Imagine you are creating a D shape in front of your body with the bar.

For a Change: Try this in reverse. Lock your shoulder blades into your back. Lift the bar in a sweeping arc out in front of your body up to chest height. Bring the bar straight in toward your chest. Keep your elbows out to the side and no higher than shoulder height. Keep the bar close to your body as you lower to starting position.

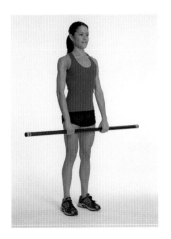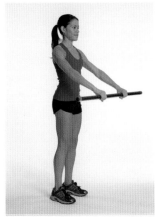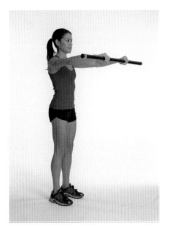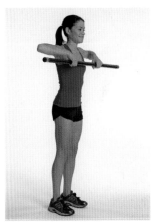

Reverse Wave

Tip: As you lift the bar, focus on keeping your shoulders down and back.

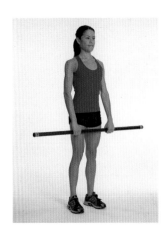

Shoulder External Rotation

The Focus: Rotator Cuff

The Setup: Lie on one side with your head either resting on your arm or propped up in the palm of your hand. Keep your shoulders, and hips in one line, with your navel pulled in toward your spine. Rest your top elbow on your waist and bend it into a 90-degree angle. Hold one end of the Body Bar in your top hand using an overhand grip. Let the other end of the bar rest on the floor in front of your feet.

The Move: Keep your elbow firmly pressed into your waist. In a sweeping motion, lift your hand out and up until it is slightly higher than hip height. Hold for a moment and slowly lower back to starting position.

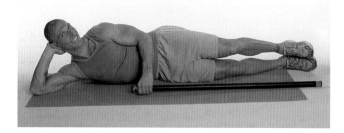 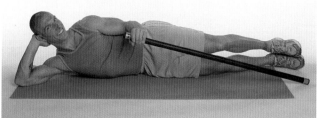

For a Change: Try this with a shorter-than-classic 4-foot bar and hold the bar in the center.

Tips: Be sure that your body does not roll forward and back as you do this exercise. Keep your wrists straight and strong.

Biceps

Biceps Curl

The Focus: Biceps

The Setup: Begin in Natural Standing Position. Hold the Body Bar at your hips with an underhand grip, your hands shoulder width apart. Keep your elbows pinned tightly to your sides and slightly bent, directly under your shoulders.

The Move: Lock your shoulder blades into your back. Flex your elbows and curl the Body Bar up toward your shoulders. Hold for a moment and slowly lower to starting position.

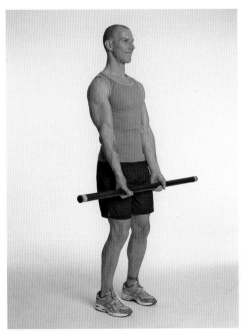 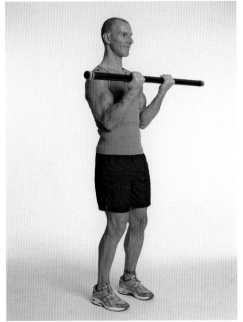

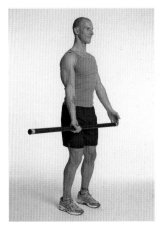

To Make It Tougher: Try an assisted single-arm biceps curl. Hold the middle of the Body Bar at your hips with an underhand grip. This will be the working arm. Lightly support the end of the bar with your other hand. Lock your shoulder blades into your back. Flex your elbow and curl the bar up toward your shoulders. Hold for a moment and slowly lower to starting position.

Tips: The position of your shoulders and elbows should be the same throughout the exercise. Concentrate on your core as you lift the bar in front of your body. Be sure to stand upright and keep your upper torso still. Avoid rocking backward to lift the bar. Either version of

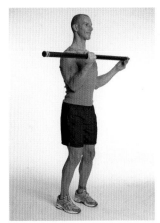

Assisted Single-Arm Biceps Curl

the biceps curl can be done with an overhand grip, an exercise called a Reverse Curl, which puts extra emphasis on the forearms.

Preacher Curl

The Focus: Biceps

The Setup: Begin in Natural Standing Position. Hold the Body Bar at your hips with an underhand grip, your hands shoulder width apart. Lower into a squat position and rest the bottom of your upper arm (just above the elbow) on your knees. Extend your elbows fully.

The Move: Lock your shoulder blades into your back. Flex your elbows and curl the Body Bar up toward your shoulders. Hold for a moment and slowly lower to starting position.

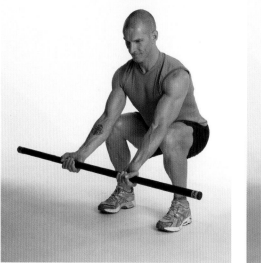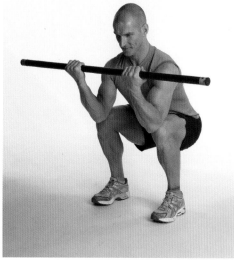

Tips: Keep your abdominal muscles engaged and your shoulder blades locked into your back.

Triceps

Lying Overhead Triceps Extension

The Focus: Triceps

The Setup: Lie on your back on the floor or a platform. Keep both feet resting squarely on the floor in front of you. Pull your navel in toward your spine. Hold the Body Bar with an overhand grip, your hands slightly closer than shoulder width apart, directly above your forehead.

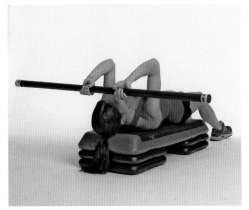 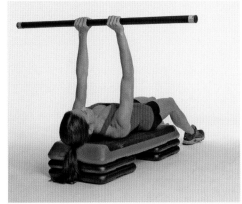

The Move: Bend your elbows and lower the bar to just behind your head. Slowly push up to starting position.

For a Change: Try this exercise standing. Begin in Natural Standing Position. Hold the Body Bar above your head with an overhand grip, your hands slightly closer than shoulder width apart. Keep your elbows close to your head. Bend your elbows and lower the bar as far as possible with good control. Slowly push up to starting position.

Tips: The position of your shoulders and elbows should be the same throughout this exercise. Don't let your elbows drift away from each other. Imagine you are holding a volleyball between them. Give your abs extra attention with this exercise to avoid hyperextension of the lower back.

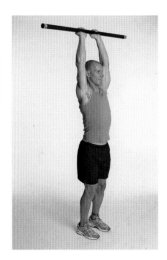

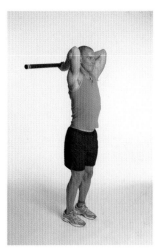

Standing Triceps Extension

Triceps Dip

The Focus: Triceps

The Setup: Begin sitting on the edge of a platform with your knees bent and feet resting squarely on the floor in front of you. Rest the Body Bar evenly across your lap. Hold on to the platform at your sides with your fingers facing forward. Lock your shoulder blades into your back. Push your palms into the platform and slide your hips forward just off the platform's edge.

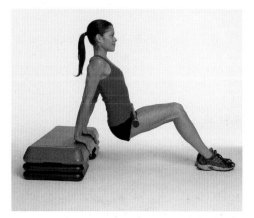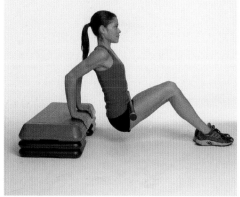

The Move: Bend your elbows and lower your hips toward the floor. Drive your palms into the platform to straighten your arms and return to starting position.

To Make It Easier: Bring your feet closer to your body.

To Make It Tougher: Step your feet farther away from your body.

Tips: With this exercise there is a heightened tendency to shrug the shoulders. Pay extra attention to keeping your shoulder blades locked into your back and your neck long. Don't let your elbows drift away from each other while doing this exercise.

Core

The Core Connection: The core is our center, our source of power. Without it, we would not have the means of supporting any other movement. It is what stabilizes us—our spines, from the very top to the lowest parts, and all the things in between both big and small. It transfers energy from muscle to muscle and is what coordinates our

Wonder Bar

Wondering . . . How to get really strong, tight, ripple-ridden abs? Try any of these abdominal exercises on a Bosu. It will allow for a bigger range of motion, as well as a balance challenge. We love it.

upper and lower bodies. Without its permission, our arms would not be allowed to carry with assuredness nor our legs to steadily transport us.

Straight-Arm Plank

The Focus: Core, Shoulders, Hip and Knee Stability

The Setup: Kneel behind a platform with the Body Bar across it. Hold the Body Bar with an overhand grip, your hands wider than shoulder width apart. Keep your wrists straight and strong. Draw your navel in toward your spine and straighten your legs so that your body is in a straight line from your head to your toes.

The Move: Hold this position.

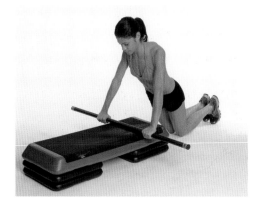 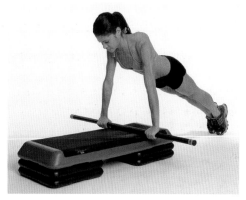

To Make It Easier: Hold the plank position on your knees.

To Make It Tougher: Try lifting one leg off the floor.

Tips: Be sure that your chin is off your chest and your hips are not sagging or up in a pike position. Either of these form breaks will compromise the benefits of this exercise.

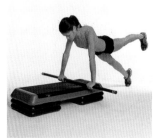

Straight-Arm Plank with One Leg Off Floor

Plank with Knee Tuck

The Focus: Core, Shoulders, Hip and Knee Stability, Hip Flexion

The Setup: Kneel behind your platform with the Body Bar across it. Hold the Body Bar with an overhand grip, your hands wider than shoulder width apart. Keep your wrists straight and strong. Draw your navel in toward your spine and straighten your legs so that your body is in a straight line from your head to your toes.

The Move: Draw one knee toward your chest, keeping that foot off the floor. Hold for a moment and return to starting position. Repeat this motion one leg at a time or alternating legs.

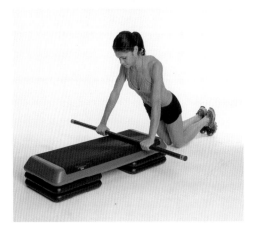 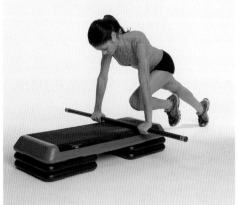

To Make It Easier: Rest the foot of the tucked knee lightly on the floor.

Plank with Hip Extension

The Focus: Core, Shoulders, Hip and Knee Stability, Hip Flexion

The Setup: Kneel behind your platform with the Body Bar across it. Hold the Body Bar with an overhand grip, your hands wider than shoulder width apart. Keep your wrists straight and strong. Draw your navel in toward your spine and straighten your legs so that you are in a straight line from your head to your toes.

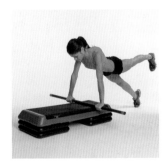

The Move: Lift one foot off the floor up to hip height. Hold for a moment, and lower back to starting position. Repeat this motion one leg at a time or alternating legs.

To Make It Easier: Rest the foot of the tucked knee lightly on the floor.

Running Plank

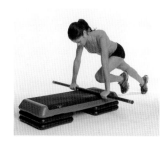

The Focus: Core, Shoulders, Hip and Knee Stability, Hip Flexion, Power and Quickness

The Setup: Begin in a straight-arm plank position with the Body Bar across the platform. Draw one knee in toward your chest. Keep that foot off the floor. Contract your abdominals in tightly.

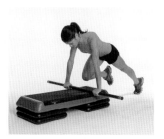

The Move: Quickly switch legs by pushing off the back foot and driving the knee toward the chest. At the same time, reach the other foot back to starting position to support your body.

To Make It Easier: Rest your front foot lightly on the floor.

To Make It Tougher: Make your run into a sprint. Increase the speed of the exercise.

Abdominal Crunch

The Focus: Rectus Abdominus (the Six-Pack)

The Setup: Lie on your back with your knees bent and your feet resting squarely on the floor in front of you. Hold the Body Bar cradled in your arms over your chest.

The Move: Pull your navel in toward your spine as you contract your abdominals. Draw your lower rib cage toward your hips, peeling your shoulder blades off the floor. Keep your chin off your chest and focus on the ceiling. At the peak of the contraction you should feel your lower back pressing into the floor. Hold for a moment and slowly return to starting position.

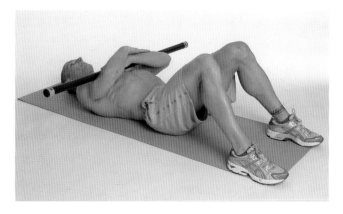
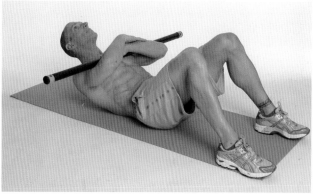

To Make It Easier: Hold the Body Bar with an underhand grip just above your hips, your hands shoulder width apart.

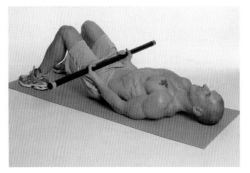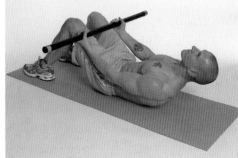

Abdominal Crunch with Underhand Grip

To Make It Tougher: Hold the Body Bar with an overhand grip at the base of your skull, your hands shoulder width apart. Allow your head to rest on the bar.

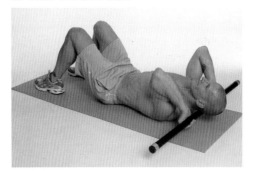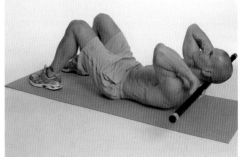

Abdominal Crunch with Body Bar at Head

Tips: As you contract your abs, exhale. Imagine flattening out your abs to squeeze the air out of your lungs.

Roll Down

The Focus: Rectus Abdominus, Transverse Abdominus, Lower Back

The Setup: Begin seated tall on the floor with your heels resting on the floor in front of you and your knees slightly bent. Hold the Body Bar with an overhand grip, your hands shoulder width apart, and extend your elbows above your forehead. Keep your elbows unlocked.

The Move: Slowly tuck the pelvis under, draw the abs in, creating a curve in the spine, and roll down one vertebra at a time until you are lying flat on the floor. As you roll down, allow your chin to drop to your chest and keep your arms extended. Imagine creating a C shape with the bar. Tuck your chin to your chest and contract your abs as you push the bar up through the same C shape to starting position, above your forehead.

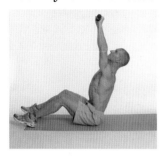 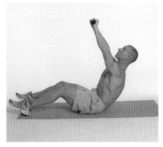 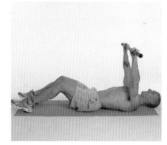

To Make It Easier: Begin with the bar at your knees. As you roll down, slide the bar down your thighs to your hips.

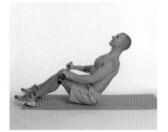 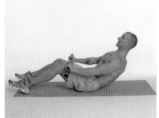 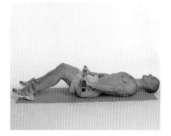

Roll Down, Beginning with Bar at Knees

Tip: At the beginning of the exercise, imagine reaching your tailbone and your shoulder blades toward each other.

Abdominal Crunch with Chest Press

The Focus: Rectus Abdominus, Pectorals, Anterior Deltoids, Triceps

The Setup: Lie on your back on a platform with both feet resting squarely on the floor in front of you. Hold the Body Bar just above your chest with an overhand grip, your hands wider than shoulder width apart. Keep your elbows directly under your fists.

The Move: Pull your navel in toward your spine as you contract your abdominals. As you draw your lower rib cage toward your hips and peel your shoulder blades off the floor, press the bar straight up to the ceiling. Keep your chin off your chest and focus on the ceiling. At the peak of the contraction you should feel you lower back pressing into the floor. Hold for a moment, and slowly lower your body and the bar to starting position.

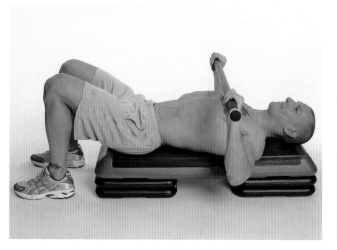 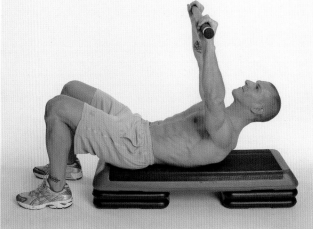

Tips: During the crunch, exhale as you contract your abs. Imagine flattening out your abs to squeeze the air out of your lungs.

Abdominal Crunch with Pullover

The Focus: Rectus Abdominus, Latissimus Dorsi, Pectorals, Posterior Deltoids

The Setup: Lie on your back on a platform with both feet resting squarely on the floor in front of you. Hold the Body Bar above your chest with an overhand grip, your hands shoulder width apart. Keep your elbows slightly bent.

The Move: Slowly lower the bar in an arc over your head toward the floor behind you until you feel a comfortable stretch at your sides and in your abs. Hold for a moment and slowly bring the bar back in the same arc to a straight-arm position over your chest. Pull your navel in toward your spine as you contract your abdominals. Draw your lower rib cage to your hips, peeling your shoulder blades off the floor. Keep your chin off your chest and focus on the ceiling. At the peak of the contraction you should feel your lower back pressing into the floor. Hold for a moment and slowly return to starting position.

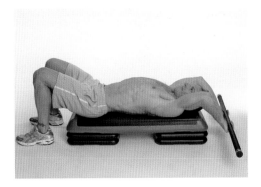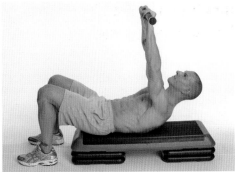

To Make It Easier: After doing the pullover, bring the bar forward to your thighs and curl up from there.

Tips: As you lower the bar behind your head, pull your navel in toward your spine to avoid hyperextending your lower back. During the crunch, exhale as you contract your abs. Imagine flattening out your abs to squeeze the air out of your lungs.

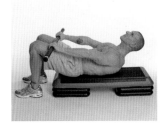

Abdominal Crunch with Pullover, with Bar at Thighs

Side Crunch

The Focus: Obliques, Transverse Abdominus, Rectus Abdominus

The Setup: Lie on the floor on your back with your knees bent over your hips at a 90-degree angle. Grasp the Body Bar underneath your knees and rest your head lightly in your hands. Contract your abs and pull your shoulder blades off the floor. Keep your chin off your chest.

The Move: Bring one elbow and one end of the bar together on one side. Hold for a moment and return to starting position. Repeat on the same side or alternate sides.

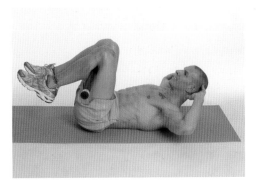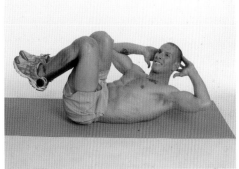

Tip: Imagine that you are trying to hold a piece of paper between your elbow and the bar.

Abdominal Crunch with Single-Arm Chest Press

The Focus: Rectus Abdominus, Obliques, Pectoral Muscles, Anterior Deltoids, Triceps

The Setup: Lie on the floor on your back with your knees bent and both feet resting squarely on the floor in front of you. Pull your navel in toward your spine. Hold the Body Bar just above your chest with an overhand grip, your hands slightly wider than shoulder width apart.

The Move: Contract your abs. Curl and rotate your torso, bringing one shoulder blade off the floor and extending fully through that arm until it is straight above your chest. Slowly lower to starting position. Repeat on the same side or alternate from side to side.

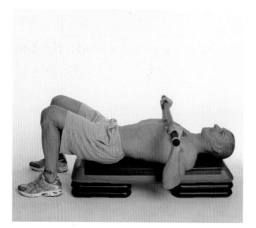 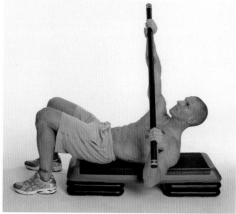

To Make It Tougher: Bring the opposite foot to the hand of the extended arm.

Tips: Exhale as you contract. Inhale as you lower your shoulder blade to the floor.

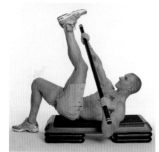

Abdominal Crunch with Single-Arm Chest Press to Opposite Foot

Bicycle Crunch

The Focus: Transverse Abdominus, Rectus Abdominus, Obliques

The Setup: Lie on the floor on your back with your knees bent over your hips at a 90-degree angle. Hold the Body Bar cradled in your arms over your chest. Contract your abs and pull your shoulder blades off the floor. Keep your chin off your chest.

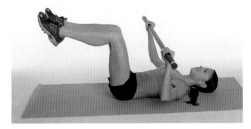 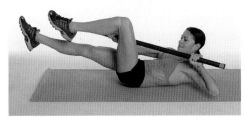

The Move: Extend one leg fully up to a 45-degree angle from the floor while drawing your other knee toward your chest. At the same time, rotate your torso, pushing the opposite elbow toward the inner thigh of your bent leg.

To Make It Easier: Try this exercise holding the bar directly over your navel. As you extend one leg, push the end of the bar toward the outside of that knee. Your elbow should touch your hip.

Tips: Keep the extended leg strong. Make sure the knee above the hip does not bend over your chest. This form break will make this move less effective.

Hip Crossover

The Focus: Rectus Abdominus

The Setup: Lie on the floor on your back with your knees bent directly over your hips. Grasp the Body Bar underneath your knees. Extend your arms directly out to the sides with your palms facing down.

The Move: Slowly twist your lower body to one side until the end of the Body Bar lightly touches the floor. In one smooth motion, twist back through the starting position to the opposite side.

Tip: Exhale with the effort.

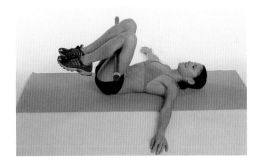 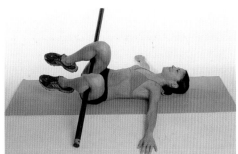

Reverse Crunch

The Focus: Rectus Abdominus

The Setup: Lie on the floor on your back with your knees bent over your hips. Hold the Body Bar directly above your shoulders with an overhand grip, your hands shoulder width apart.

The Move: Contract your abs. Curl your hips off the floor and draw your knees toward your elbows. Hold for a moment and slowly crunch down to starting position.

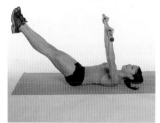

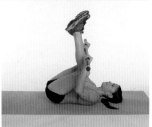

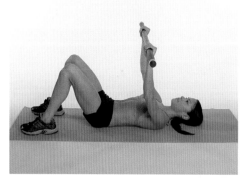

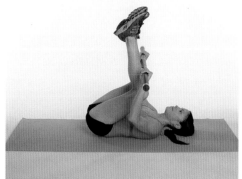

To Make It Tougher: Begin with your legs extended over your hips, either straight or with your knees slightly bent. Lower your legs to about 45 degrees, maintaining a neutral spine. Bend your knees and draw them in toward your elbows, curling your hips off the floor. Straighten your legs and try to touch your shins to the bar. Slowly roll your hips down to the floor.

Tip: Focus extra attention on pulling your navel in toward your spine to avoid hyperextension of your back as you lower your legs out to the 45-degree position.

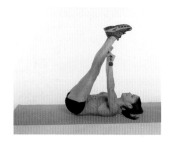

**Reverse Crunch
Advanced**

Reverse Crunch with Bar Behind Knees

The Focus: Rectus Abdominus

The Setup: Lie on the floor on your back with your knees bent and your feet off the floor. Grasp the Body Bar underneath your knees.

The Move: Contract your abs. Curl your hips off the floor and draw your knees toward your chin. Hold for a moment and slowly curl back to starting position until your feet touch the floor lightly.

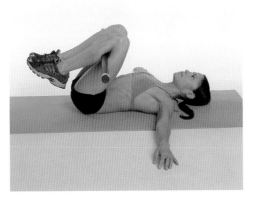 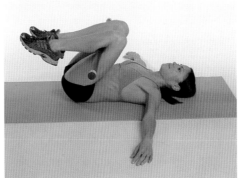

To Make It Tougher: Rest your head lightly in your fingers and curl your upper and lower torso up at the same time.

Full-Body Crunch

The Focus: Rectus Abdominus, Hip Flexor

The Setup: Lie on the floor on your back with your knees bent over your hips. Hold the Body Bar directly above your forehead with an overhand grip, your hands shoulder width apart. Keep your forearms parallel to each other.

The Move: Contract your abs. Pull your hips and shoulder blades off the floor, coming into a tight, ball-like contraction. Bring the bar just above your knees. Hold for a moment and slowly lower back to starting position.

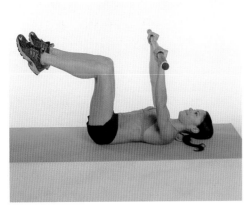 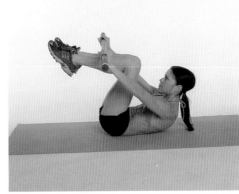

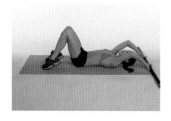

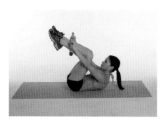

**Full-Body Crunch
Advanced**

To Make It Tougher: Begin with your toes lightly touching the floor in front of you and your knuckles lightly touching the floor behind your head. Keep your elbows slightly bent. At the top of the contraction, try to touch the bar to your ankles.

Tips: Keep your shoulder blades locked into your back and your neck long throughout this exercise.

Kayaker

The Focus: Entire Shoulder Girdle, Core Muscles

The Setup: Begin in a V-sit position. In this position, your upper body is tilted back slightly, your feet are off the floor, and your knees are bent. Lift out of your lower back, working to keep your torso long. Hold the Body Bar at shoulder height with a wide overhand grip.

The Move: Reach one arm straight out beyond your knees as if you were reaching ahead of you to dip a paddle in the water. Lower the end of the bar to a few inches off the floor. Pull that end of the bar until it is at your side while allowing your other arm to reach out beyond your other knee. Imagine that you are drawing an egg shape on either side of your body with the ends of the bar. Work to create a fluid, continuous motion.

To Make It Easier: Let your feet rest squarely on the floor in front of you. You can also draw smaller circles with the ends of the Body Bar.

Tips: Think of lifting through the chest and pushing your tailbone down and back into the floor. This should help to maintain the natural curve of your lower back. Imagine that you are actually paddling a kayak.

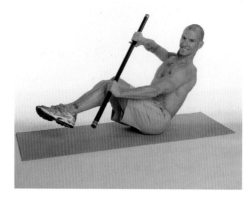

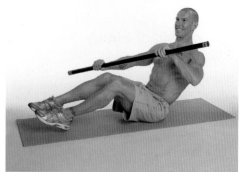

Lower-Back Extension

The Focus: Lower Back

The Setup: Lie facedown with your arms extended fully in front of you with your palms down and your wrists resting on the Body Bar. Keep your neck long. You should be looking down at the floor.

The Move: Roll the Body Bar toward you as you pull your shoulders blades down your back, and peel your chest off the floor. Hold for a moment and slowly lower to starting position.

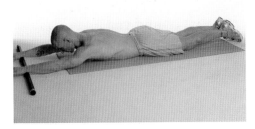 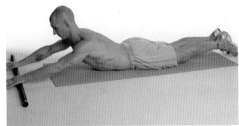

To Make It Tougher: Try lifting one or both legs as you peel your chest off the floor.

Tip: Be sure to keep your arms extended throughout this exercise.

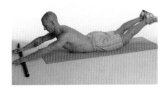

Lower-Back Extension with Both Legs Off Floor

Multitask Exercises

Life is one fluid, continuous motion. By practicing multitask exercises, we train our bodies to integrate our movements gracefully and efficiently.

Chest Press and Pullover Arc

The Focus: Latissimus Dorsi, Rear Deltoids, Upper Back, Pectorals, Triceps, Serratus

The Setup: Lie on your back on a platform with both feet resting squarely on the floor in front of you. Pull your navel in toward your spine. Hold the Body Bar above your chest with an overhand grip, your hands shoulder width apart. Keep your elbows slightly bent.

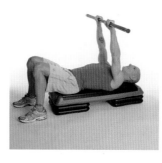 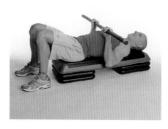 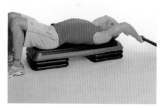

The Move: Slowly lower the Body Bar to the middle of your chest. Press the bar back up to starting position and slowly lower it in an arc over your head toward the floor behind you until you feel a comfortable stretch at your sides and in your abs. Hold for a moment and slowly bring the bar back in the same arc to a straight-arm position over your chest.

To Make It Tougher: Try this exercise unilaterally. Be sure to have mastered the bilateral movement and feel completely comfortable moving on. This variation will be a much bigger challenge for your shoulder stabilizers. Hold the middle of the Body Bar in one hand with an overhand grip.

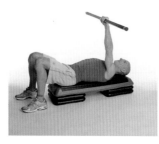 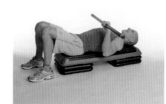 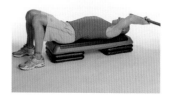

Chest Press with Pullover

Tips: The bend in your elbows should not change throughout this exercise. Give your abs extra attention to avoid hyperextension of the lower back. Keep your wrists straight and strong.

Upright Row with Shoulder Press

The Focus: Anterior Deltoids, Trapezius, Biceps, Triceps

The Setup: Begin in Natural Standing Position. Hold the Body Bar at your hips with an overhand grip, your hands shoulder width apart.

The Move: Lift the bar, keeping it close to your body, until your elbows are at shoulder height. Tuck your elbows under the bar and push the bar toward the ceiling until your arms are fully extended but not locked. Reverse the motion to lower the bar to starting position.

To Make It Tougher: Rotate your torso to one side as you push the bar up to the ceiling. This variation will challenge your core stability.

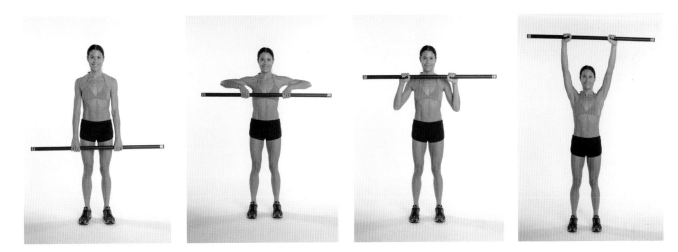

Tips: Keep your neck long. Imagine driving your shoulder blades down your back as you press the bar overhead. Concentrate on pulling your navel tightly in toward your spine, especially if you are adding a rotation to the shoulder press.

Front Step-Up with Shoulder Press

The Focus: Quadriceps, Hamstrings, Gluteals, Anterior Deltoids, Trapezius, Triceps

The Setup: Begin with one foot on the floor and one foot on the platform in front of you. Hold the Body Bar at shoulder height with an overhand grip, your hands slightly wider than shoulder width apart.

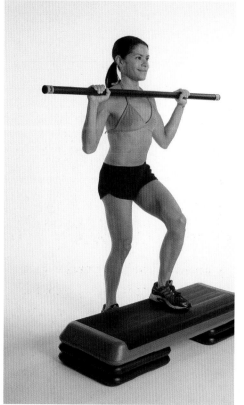 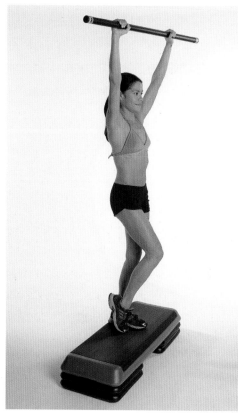

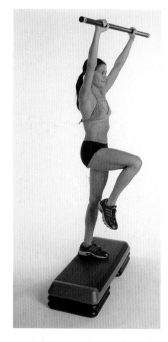

Front Step-Up with Shoulder Press and Knee Lift

The Move: Push into the platform with the raised leg and step up onto it. As you stand, push the bar toward the ceiling until your arms are fully extended but not locked. As you lower to starting position, lower the bar to shoulder height.

To Make It Tougher: Lift your knee to hip height or higher as you press the bar to the ceiling.

Tip: Think of climbing up a step and putting something up on a shelf.

Squat with Shoulder Press

The Focus: Quadriceps, Gluteals, Hamstrings, Anterior Deltoids, Trapezius, Triceps

The Setup: Begin in Natural Standing Position. Hold the Body Bar at shoulder height with an overhand grip, your hands slightly wider than shoulder width apart.

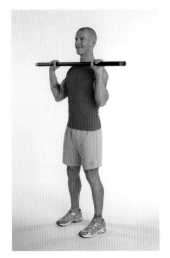
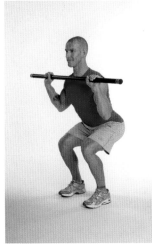
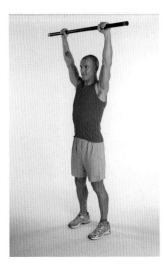

The Move: Bend your knees and push your hips back as you lower your body as far as you can, creating up to a 90-degree angle at the knees. You should feel your weight over your ankles. Keep your chin lifted off your chest and your focus out in front of you. Imagine pushing the ground away from you as you stand up to starting position. In one smooth motion as you stand, push the bar toward the ceiling until your arms are fully extended but not locked. As you sit back into the squat position, lower the bar back to shoulder height.

To Make It Tougher: Rotate your torso about 45 degrees as you press. Don't bring your knees and hips with you as you rotate; keep them facing forward. You can increase the difficulty of this exercise by performing it unilaterally. This variation will put more emphasis on shoulder stabilization. Hold the Body Bar in the middle with an overhand grip and your elbow out to the side. Push the bar in an arc toward the ceiling until your arm is fully extended but not locked, straight above your shoulder. Hold for a moment and slowly lower in the same arc to starting position.

Tips: Never drop the bar below shoulder height. Always keep your elbows right underneath the bar.

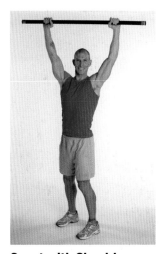

Squat with Shoulder Press and Rotation

Clean-and-Press

The Focus: Hamstrings, Gluteals, Lower Back, Anterior Deltoids, Trapezius, Triceps, Biceps

The Setup: Begin in Natural Standing Position. Hold the Body Bar at your hips with an overhand grip, your hands wider than shoulder width apart.

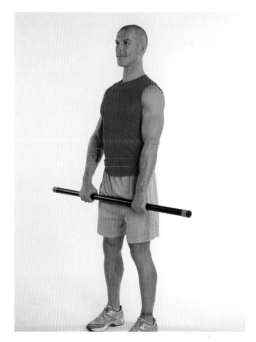 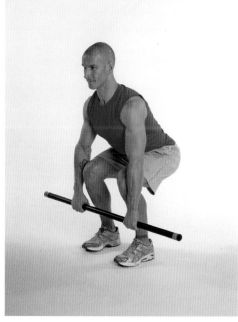

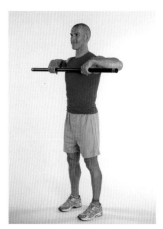 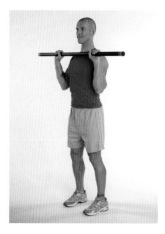 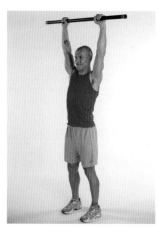

The Move: Bend your knees, push your hips back, and slide the bar down your thighs as if you wanted to put the bar on the floor. You should be in a squat position with the bar slightly lower than knee height. Keep your shoulder blades locked into your back, your chin lifted off your chest, and your focus forward. You should feel most of your weight over your ankles. Drive your feet into the floor as you push your hips forward. As you stand, pull the bar in a straight line from the floor to your shoulders. Tuck your elbows under the bar and push the bar toward the ceiling until your arms are fully extended but not locked. Reverse the motion to get down to squat position.

To Make It Tougher: Do a calf raise as you extend your arms in the shoulder press.

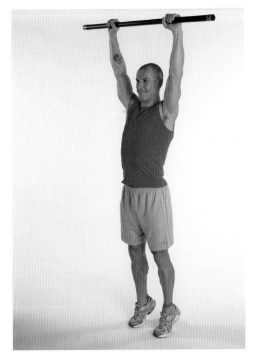 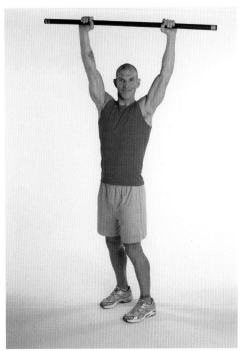

Clean-and-Press with Calf Raise   **Clean-and-Press with Rotation**

To Make It Even Tougher: Rotate your torso about 45 degrees as you press. Don't bring your knees and hips with you as you rotate; keep them facing forward.

Tips: The bar should travel in a straight line from the squat position up to your shoulders. Avoid the tendency to swing the bar out away from you to get to shoulder height.

Reverse Wave with Squat

The Focus: Quadriceps, Gluteals, Hamstrings, Anterior Deltoids, Biceps

The Setup: Begin in Natural Standing Position. Hold the Body Bar at your hips with an overhand grip, your hands shoulder width apart.

The Move: Lock your shoulder blades into your back. Bend your knees and push your hips back as you lower your body as far as you can, creating up to a 90-degree angle at the knees, while lifting the bar in a sweeping arc out in front of you up to shoulder height. You should feel your weight over your ankles. Keep your chin lifted off your chest and your focus out in front of you. As you come out of the squat, draw the bar in toward your chest and back down close to your body to starting position.

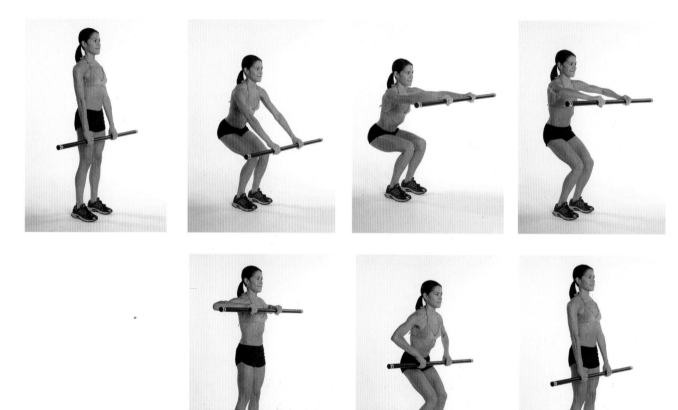

Tip: Keep your elbows above the bar and at about shoulder height as you draw the bar in toward your chest.

Stirring the Pot with a Squat

The Focus: Quadriceps, Hamstrings, Gluteals, Anterior Deltoids, Medial Deltoids, Posterior Deltoids, Upper Back, Core Stability

The Setup: Begin in Natural Standing Position. Hold the middle of the Body Bar vertically in both hands directly in front of your body.

The Move: Lock your shoulder blades into your back. As you lower your body in a squat, draw circles with the Body Bar as if you were stirring a pot.

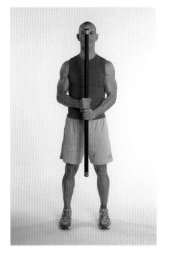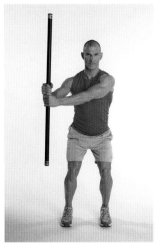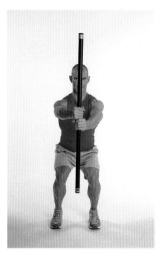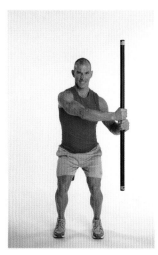

Tips: The bar should be farthest away from you at the bottom of your squat. Because your body is counterbalanced with the Body Bar during this move, work to keep your upper body upright during the squat. Beware of shrugging your shoulders. Keep your neck long throughout this movement. Don't forget to do equal sets in both directions with your arms!

Rainbow Squat

The Focus: Quadriceps, Hamstrings, Gluteals, Anterior Deltoids, Medial Deltoids, Posterior Deltoids, Latissimus Dorsi, Core Stability

The Setup: Begin in Natural Standing Position. Hold the middle of the Body Bar vertically in both hands directly in front of your body.

The Move: Rotate your torso to one side as you lower your body into a squat. Lightly touch the bar on the floor. As you push out of the

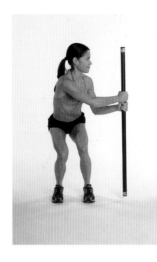 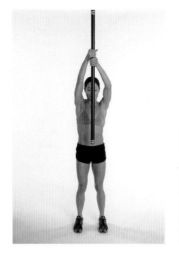 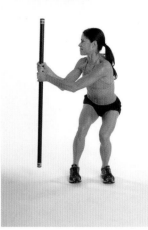

squat, lift both arms up in a rainbow arc over your body to repeat on the other side.

Tip: Pay extra attention to keeping your core stabilized throughout this move.

Dead Lift to Pendulum

The Focus: Hamstrings, Gluteals, Lower Back, Medial Deltoids

The Setup: Begin in Natural Standing Position. Hold the Body Bar at your hips with an extra-wide and relaxed overhand grip. Keep your wrists straight and strong.

The Move: Bend your knees, push your hips back, and slide the bar down your thighs as if you wanted to put the bar on the floor. You should be in a squat position with the bar slightly lower than knee

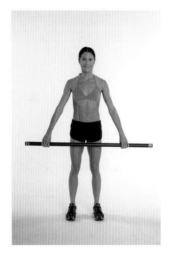 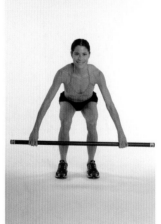 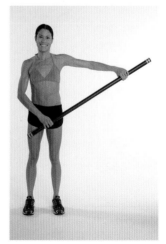

height. Keep your shoulder blades locked into your back, holding your back flat. Keep your chin lifted off your chest and your focus forward. You should feel most of your weight over your ankles. Drive your feet into the floor as you push your hips forward to stand up to starting position. As you stand, lift the bar out to the side in a sweeping arc up to shoulder height. Hold for a moment and slowly lower the arm in the same arc as you sit back into the squat position. Try this exercise either working one arm at a time or alternating from one side to the other.

Tips: As you lift the bar out to the side, loosen your grip slightly so that your wrists stay in a neutral position. At that point you should be holding the bar primarily with your thumb and index finger.

Modified Single-Leg Dead Lift with Narrow-Grip Row

The Focus: Hamstrings, Gluteals, Lower Back, Upper Back, Posterior Deltoids, Core Stability

The Setup: Begin in Natural Standing Position. Hold the Body Bar at your hips with an underhand grip, your hands shoulder width apart.

The Move: Shift your weight to one leg. This will be your working leg. Keep your legs straight but your knees soft. Hinge at the hips to a 90-degree angle and slide the bar down your thighs to knee height while reaching the nonworking leg straight back toward the wall behind you. Keep your back flat. You should feel most of your weight over the ankle of the working leg. Using your back muscles, pull the bar up to just below your navel. Keep your elbows tucked in and

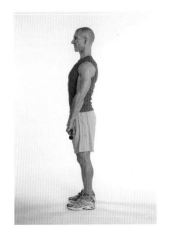 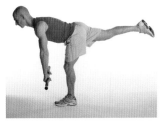 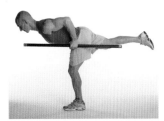

close to the sides of your body throughout the exercise. Hold for a moment and slowly release as you push up to starting position.

To Make It Tougher: Do a single-arm row. With the arm opposite the working leg, hold the middle of the bar with an overhand grip at your side. Keep your elbow close to your body and pull your hand back to your hip.

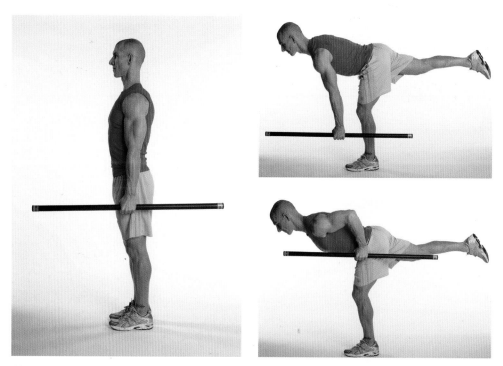

Single-Arm Single-Leg Modified Dead Lift with Narrow-Grip Row

Tip: As you pull the bar, squeeze your shoulder blades together as if you were trying to hold a pencil between them.

Squat Thrust

The Focus: Full-Body Integration

The Setup: Begin in Natural Standing Position. Hold the Body Bar at your hips with an overhand grip, your hands wider than shoulder width apart. Stand about 3 to 6 inches away from the end of the platform.

The Move: Squat and lower the bar across the end of the platform with your chest directly over the bar. Push into the platform and jump your feet back into a push-up position. Jump your feet forward

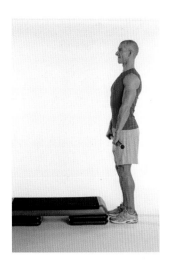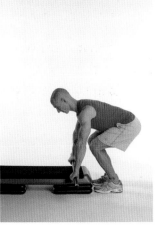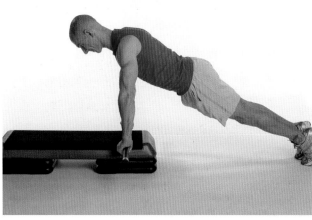

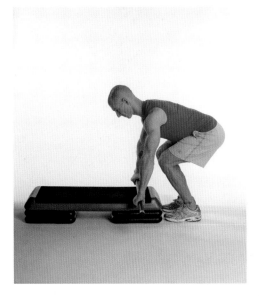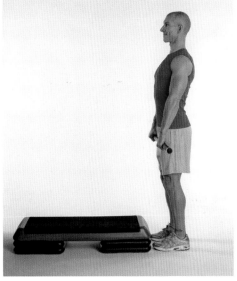

and underneath you. Drive your feet into the floor as you push your hips forward to return to starting position with the Body Bar at your hips.

To Make It Tougher: Make this exercise into a squat thrust push-up. When you are in a straight-arm plank position over the platform, lower your chest to the bar and push back up before jumping your feet forward to stand.

Tip: Brace your core so your hips don't sag.

Ultimate Full-Body Combo

The Focus: Full-Body Integration

The Setup: Begin in Natural Standing Position. Hold the Body Bar at your hips with an overhand grip, your hands wider than shoulder width apart. Stand about 3 to 6 inches away from the end of the platform.

The Move: Squat and lower the bar across the end of the platform with your chest directly over the bar. Push into the platform and jump your feet back into a push-up position. Perform a push-up. Jump your feet forward and underneath you. Drive your feet into the floor as you push your hips forward to stand. As you come up from the squat, pull the bar in a straight line from the floor to your shoulders. Tuck your elbows under the bar. Push the bar toward the ceiling until your arms are fully extended but not locked. Lower the bar to shoulder height. In a straight line, lower the bar right back to the platform and repeat the exercise.

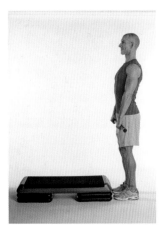 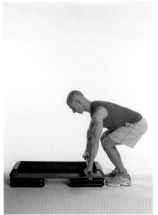 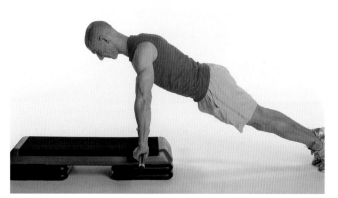

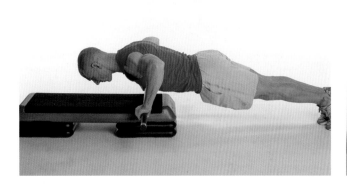 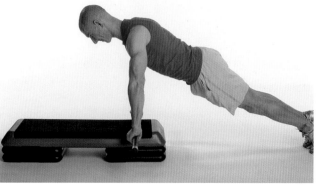

(continued on next page)

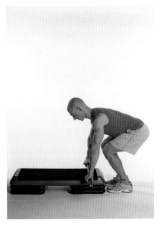 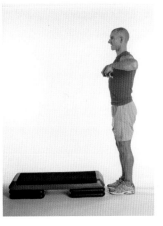 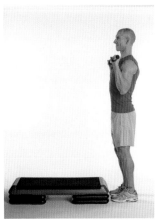 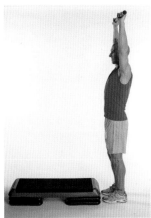

Ultimate Full Body Combo (cont)

To Make It Easier: Use a taller platform.

To Make It Tougher: Speed it up or use a lower platform, or both.

Tips: When lowering into the squat position, maintain a flat back. Keep your chin lifted off your chest and your focus forward. In the push-up position, brace your core to lock your body in a straight line from head to toe. Don't let your hips sag.

Single-Arm Row with Knee Lift

The Focus: Latissimus Dorsi, Gluteals, Hips, Quadriceps, Hamstrings

The Setup: Begin in Natural Standing Position. Hold the middle of the Body Bar with an overhand grip at your side. Step the leg on that side back approximately 3 steps. Hinge at the hips up to approximately 45 degrees and let the bar hang straight down to the floor. Rest your nonworking arm on your front thigh.

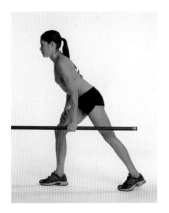

The Move: Bend your front knee and shift most of your weight to that leg. Pull the bar up to your hip, keeping your elbows tucked in and close to the sides of your body. As you pull the bar, lift the knee of the back leg to your chest. Hold for a moment. Slowly lower your arm and leg to starting position.

To Make It Tougher: Bend deeper into your standing leg. The deeper you bend that knee, the more effective this exercise.

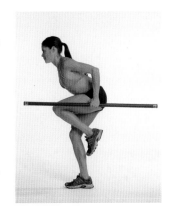

Tip: In the starting position, your body should be a straight line from the top of your head to your feet. Be sure to keep your standing leg bent.

Lunge-Twist-Press

The Focus: Quadriceps, Hamstrings, Gluteals, Anterior Deltoids, Trapezius, Triceps, Core Stability

The Setup: Begin in Natural Standing Position. Hold the Body Bar with an overhand grip at shoulder height, your hands slightly wider than shoulder width apart. Take a large step forward in a straight line. Your weight should be evenly distributed between both feet.

The Move: Bend both knees and lower directly to the floor until your knees are bent up to a 90-degree angle. Most of your weight should now be over the ankle of your front leg; your back heel will be off the floor. As you lower your body, rotate in the direction of your front leg. As you stand out of the lunge, rotate your torso back to center and push the bar toward the ceiling until your arms are fully extended but not locked. Lower the bar to shoulder height and return to starting position.

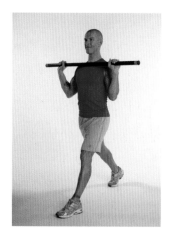 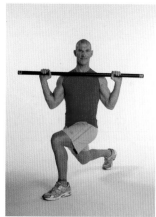 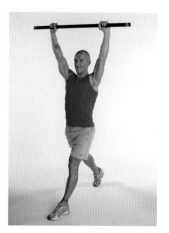

Tip: Keep your knees aligned with your toes.

Front-to-Back Lunge with Biceps Curl

The Focus: Quadriceps, Hamstrings, Gluteals, Biceps

The Setup: Begin in Natural Standing Position. Hold the Body Bar at your hips with an underhand grip, your hands shoulder width apart.

The Move: Take a step forward in a straight line. Bend both knees and lower directly to the floor until your knees are bent up to a 90-

degree angle. Most of your weight will be over the ankle of your front leg; your back heel will be off the floor. As you step, curl the Body Bar up to your shoulders. Drive your front foot into the floor to push yourself out of the lunge as you lower the bar back to your hips. Step right through starting position and step backward in a straight line, again curling the bar to your shoulders. Push into the ground with your front foot to stand, and lower the bar to starting position.

To Make It Tougher: Rotate your torso toward the front leg of the lunge as you curl the bar toward your shoulders.

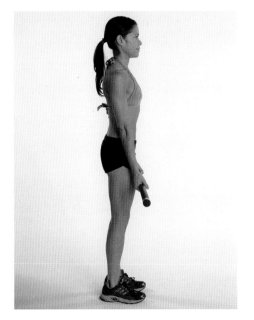
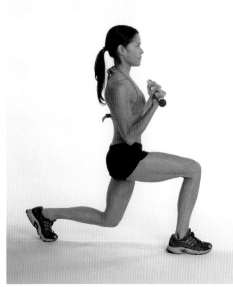
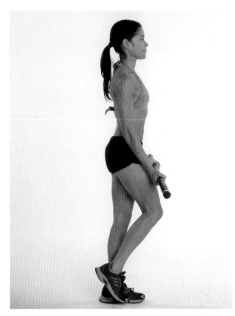
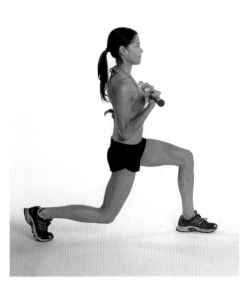

Tip: Keep your elbows pinned to your waist throughout this movement.

Reverse Lunge with Front Raise

The Focus: Quadriceps, Hamstrings, Gluteals, Anterior Deltoids

The Setup: Begin in Natural Standing Position. Hold the Body Bar at your hips with an overhand grip, your hands shoulder width apart.

The Move: Take a step backward in a straight line. Keep your body weight over the ankle of your front leg. Bend both knees and lower directly to the floor until your knees are bent up to a 90-degree angle. Most of your weight will be over the ankle of the front leg; your back heel will be off the floor. As you step back, lift the bar in a sweeping arc out in front of your body up to shoulder height. Drive your front foot into the floor to return to starting position as you lower the bar to your hips.

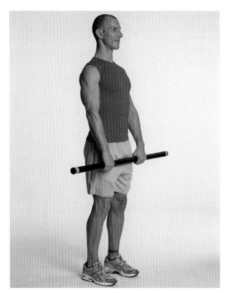 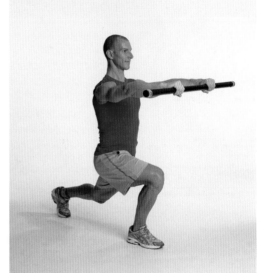

Tips: Keep your shoulder blades locked into your back and your neck long throughout this exercise.

Reverse Lunge with Single-Arm Press

The Focus: Quadriceps, Hamstrings, Gluteals, Anterior Deltoids, Trapezius, Triceps

The Setup: Begin in Natural Standing Position. Hold the middle of the Body Bar with an overhand grip at shoulder height, your elbows tucked into your sides.

The Move: With the leg farthest from the bar, take a step backward in a straight line. Keep your body weight over the ankle of your front leg. Bend both knees and lower directly to the floor until your knees are bent up to a 90-degree angle. Most of your weight will be over the ankle of your front leg; your back heel will be off the floor. As you push down into the ground with your front foot to return to starting position, press the bar up toward the ceiling. Your arm should be extended but not locked. Lower your arm as you step back into the lunge.

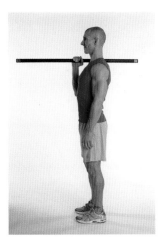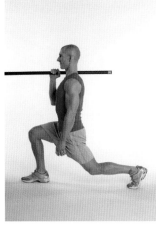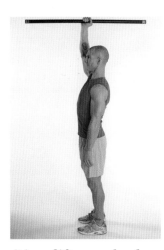

To Make It Tougher: As you return to starting position, lift your back foot off the floor, raising your knee to hip height or higher.

Tips: As you push the bar up with any type of shoulder press, imagine pushing your shoulder blades down your back, creating a long feeling in your neck. Concentrate on keeping the movement slow, smooth, and controlled.

Curtsy Lunge with Upright Row

The Focus: Quadriceps, Hamstrings, Gluteals, Anterior Deltoids, Biceps

The Setup: Begin in Natural Standing Position. Hold the Body Bar at your hips with an overhand grip, your hands shoulder width apart.

The Move: Shift your weight to one side. Step backward in a diagonal line behind your standing leg. Bend both knees and lower directly to the floor, creating up to a 90-degree angle with your front knee. Most of your weight will be over the ankle of your front foot; your back

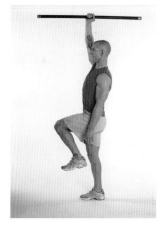

Reverse Lunge with Single-Arm Press and Knee Raise

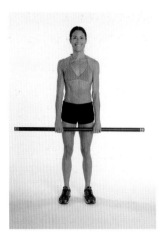
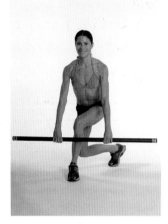
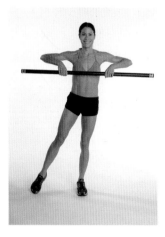

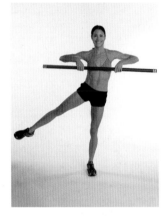

**Curtsy Lunge with
Upright Row and Kick**

heel will be off the floor. In one smooth motion, stand up to starting position and lift the bar, keeping it close to your body until your elbows are at shoulder height. Hold for a moment and slowly lower your arms and body to the curtsy position.

To Make It Tougher: To intensify this move, add the kick option. When lifting out of the lunge, shift your weight to the nonlunging leg and kick out to the side. Follow by dropping back into the lunge.

Side Lunge with Pendulum

The Focus: Quadriceps, Hamstrings, Gluteals, Medial Deltoids

The Setup: Begin in Natural Standing Position. Hold the Body Bar at your hips with an extra-wide, relaxed, overhand grip. Keep your wrists straight and strong.

The Move: Take a large step (approximately 2 to 3 feet) out to one side. Push your hips back and bend your knee, creating up to a 90-degree angle. As you step, lift the bar in a sweeping arc in the oppo-

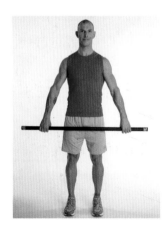
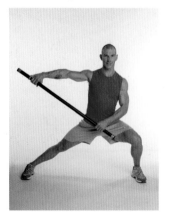
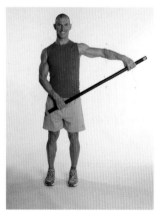

site direction up to shoulder height. Push off the floor with enough force to return your body to starting position, as you sweep the bar in an arc to the other side up to shoulder height.

Tip: Be sure to keep your chin lifted off your chest and your focus forward. Keep the lunging knee aligned with your toes and most of your weight over the ankle of the lunging leg. Throughout this move, both of your feet should face forward and your nonlunging leg should remain straight.

Shoveler

The Focus: Full-Body Integration

The Setup: Begin in Natural Standing Position. Hold the Body Bar at your hips with one hand in the middle using an underhand grip, and the other at the end of the bar using an overhand grip.

The Move: Step out to a side lunge, while reaching the Body Bar toward the ground as if you were digging something up from the earth (a hidden treasure chest full of gold would be nice). Push up from the lunge to return to starting position. As you are pushing up, create an arc with the Body Bar across your body. Imagine that you are throwing what you have just dug up off to the side. Keep the arm with the overhand grip close to your side.

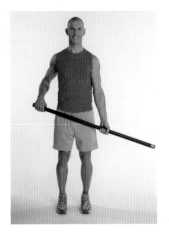 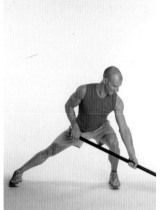 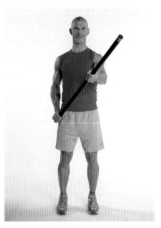 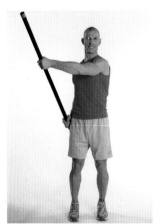

Tip: Be vigilant about keeping your abdominals engaged throughout this movement.

Wonder Bar

Wondering . . . what "plyometric" training is? It is the type of training that cultivates fast muscle fibers. Have you ever seen a sprinter bolting out at the start of a race with nimble legs churning into action? Imagine stretching out a coiled spring as far as possible and then letting it go. In the instant it takes for the spring to recoil, explosive energy is released. In the same way, a muscle is able to contract with a greater amount of strength and speed if it is first lengthened. Plyometric exercises help the muscles develop the ability to rapidly and vigorously lengthen and recoil.

Plyometric, Quickness, and Agility Exercises

Plyometric, quickness, and agility training are great ways to add intensity to your workouts. These exercises are advanced and should be attempted only if you are already active on a regular basis.

Lateral Leap

The Focus: Quadriceps, Hamstrings, Gluteals, Quickness. This move will help increase your lower body's lateral strength and stability.

The Setup: Place the Body Bar on the floor at a 90-degree angle to your body. Make sure you have ample free space on both sides of the bar. Begin in a semisquat position on one side of the bar. Keep your chin lifted off your chest and your focus forward.

The Move: Push off the foot farthest away from the bar, leaping laterally up and over the bar and landing on the opposite leg. Absorb your landing by bending your knee. Move from side to side with quickness, power, and control.

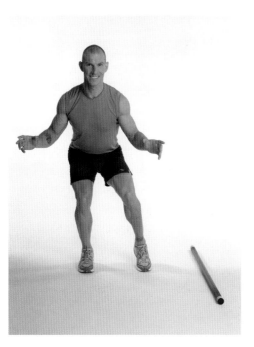
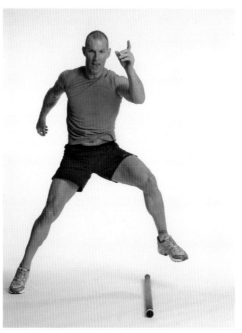
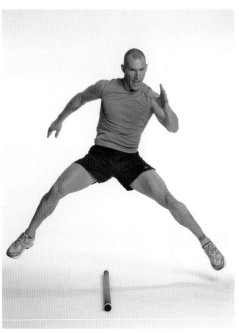
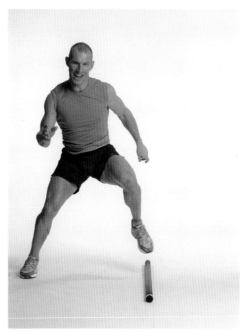

To Make It Tougher: Jump higher and wider. Deepen your landing. Accelerate the move.

Tips: Pay attention to the position of the bar with each jump. If you are new to this exercise, try the movement without the bar first.

Slalom

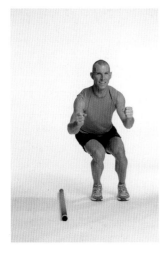

The Focus: Quadriceps, Hamstrings, Gluteals, Quickness. This move will help increase your lower body's lateral strength and stability.

The Setup: Place the Body Bar vertically on the floor. Make sure you have ample free space on both sides of the bar. Begin in a semisquat position on one side of the bar. Bring your arms out in front of you as if you were holding ski poles. Keep your chin lifted off your chest and your focus forward.

The Move: Leap laterally over the bar with both feet. Land softly by bending your knees and lowering into a semisquat position. Move from side to side with quickness and control.

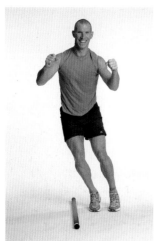
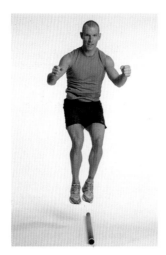
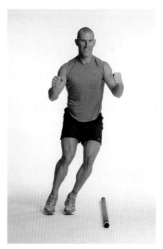
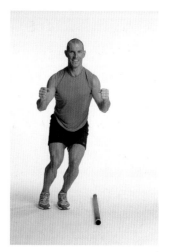

To Make It Tougher: Speed it up.

Tips: Pay attention to the position of the bar with each jump. If you are new to this exercise, try the movement without the bar first.

Split Squat Jump

The Focus: Quadriceps, Hamstrings, Gluteals, Quickness, Power. This move will help increase your lower body's strength and stability.

The Setup: Begin in a basic lunge position with the Body Bar across your shoulders.

The Move: Drive your feet into the floor, jumping up out of the lunge and switching your feet in the air. Land back in the lunge position softly.

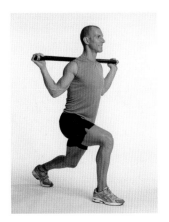 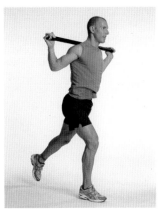 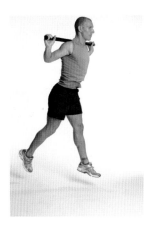 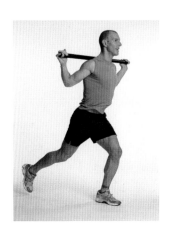

To Make It Easier: Hold the Body Bar vertically in front of you, with both hands at the top of the bar. Push down into the bar, to ease your landing.

To Make It Tougher: Increase height and speed. You can also try this movement with one foot up on a platform.

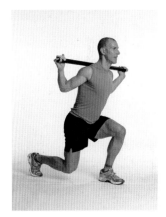

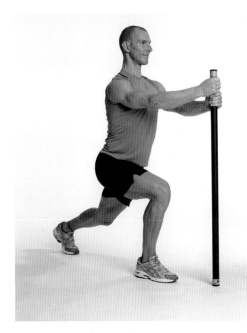

Easier Split Squat Jump

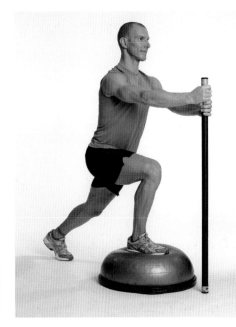

Split Squat Jump with One Foot on Platform

Tips: Give your core special attention. Imagine trying to land without making a sound.

Hot Feet on the Floor or the Bosu

The Focus: Quadriceps, Hamstrings, Gluteals, Quickness. This move will help increase your lower body's speed.

The Setup: Sit in a squat position with your feet about hip width apart and your hands out in front of you.

The Move: Drum the balls of your feet on the floor with explosive quickness.

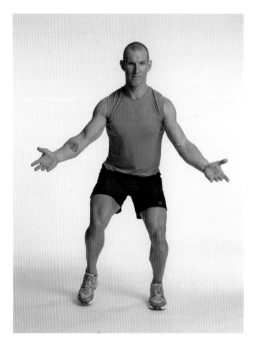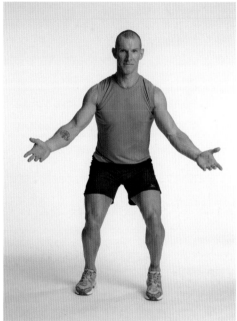

Tip: Imagine that you are barefoot on hot coals.

The Workouts

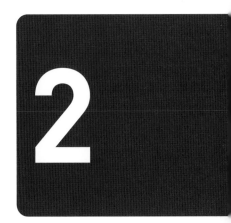

The Fundamentals

A solid foundation is at the base of anything long lasting and strong. Let the Fundamentals be your workout foundation. They will lay the basic groundwork necessary to begin with, and they will help you build good workout habits. Become a master at performing each of these exercises with correct form and technique first. Then try them in a workout. Full Body—Beginner 1, the first workout in this book, is made up of only the Fundamentals.

With regard to all the workouts in this chapter, at the end of the day, it is *your* body and the workouts are for *you*. We have equipped you with an arsenal of exercises; do not feel limited by the particular ones included in our workouts. Feel free to replace one exercise with another for the same muscle group. Variety is the means to successful progress. Simply changing the order in which you do the exercises within a workout will keep your body guessing and will keep things fresh for your mind. Try not to get stuck on always doing your favorite workout. Create new challenges for yourself and combine the workouts in different ways.

Exercises to master before beginning workouts:

Basic Squat

Front Step-Up

Basic Lunge

Modified Dead Lift

Straight-Arm Plank (start kneeling; work your way up to the full version)

Push-Up

Narrow-Grip Bent-Over Row

Chest Press

Shoulder Press

Lower-Back Extension

Side Crunch

Crunches

Full Body—Beginner 1

Time: 10–20 minutes

Props: Body Bar, platform

Drill: Do 10–15 reps of each exercise. For single-sided exercises, do a full set on each side. If you make it through this circuit and feel like you are ready to take it to the next level, go through the circuit twice or do two sets of each exercise before moving on to the next.

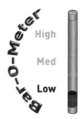

Bar-O-Meter
High
Med
Low

Straight-Arm Plank (15–60 seconds; remember: kneeling is an option)

Basic Squat

Push-Up

Basic Lunge

Narrow-Grip Bent-Over Row

Front Step-Up
(one side at a time)

Shoulder Press

Modified Dead Lift

Chest Press

Lower-Back Extension

Side Crunch

Abdominal Crunch

Warming up your muscles will get your blood circulating through them and will help prevent injuries. Warming up will also help you work harder for a longer period of time. Choose any low-intensity aerobic exercise that is convenient for you or that you particularly love. It can be anything . . . a brisk walk on a treadmill, a bike ride, a few trips up and down the stairs, or dancing to your favorite music. Go for something that will make you break a bit of a sweat.

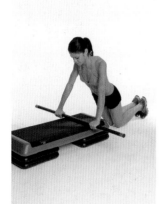

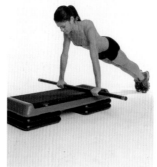

Straight-Arm Plank (15–60 seconds; remember: kneeling is an option)

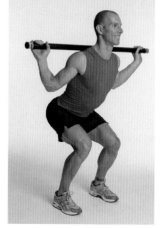

Basic Squat

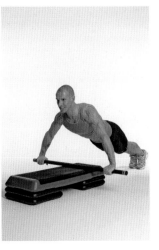

Push-Up

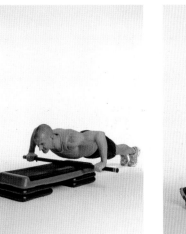

Basic Lunge

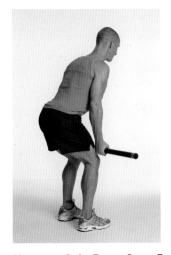

Narrow-Grip Bent-Over Row

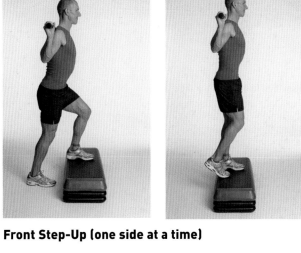

Front Step-Up (one side at a time)

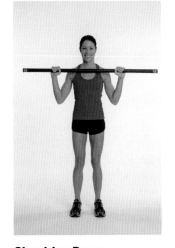

Shoulder Press

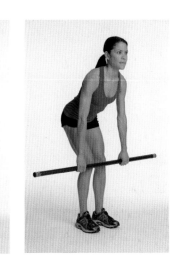

Modified Dead Lift

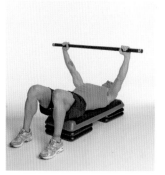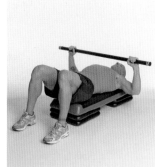

Chest Press

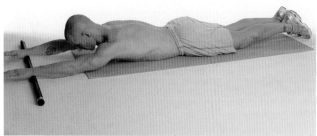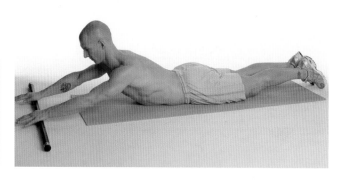

Lower-Back Extension

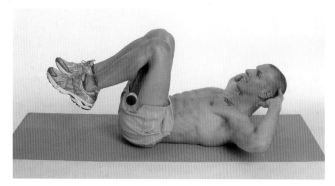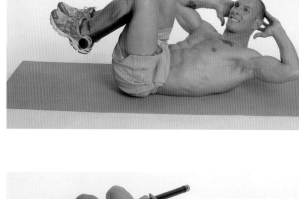

Side Crunch

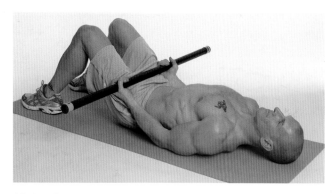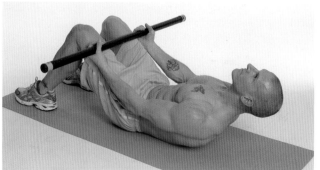

Abdominal Crunch

Full Body—Beginner 2

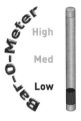

Basic Squat

Front Step-Up (one side at a time)

Standing Side Leg Lift

Modified Dead Lift

Straight-Arm Plank (15–30 seconds; remember: kneeling is an option)

Chest Press

Narrow-Grip Bent-Over Row

Shoulder Press

Rear Shoulder Extension

Straight-Arm Plank (15–30 seconds; remember: kneeling is an option)

Forward Lunge (alternating legs; use the bar for balance if necessary)

Frowning Squat

Side-Lying Inner-Thigh Lift

Lower-Back Extension

Abdominal Crunch with Single-Arm Chest Press

Abdominal Crunch (with the bar either on your hips or cradled across your chest)

Reverse Crunch with Bar Behind Knees

Build your weaknesses until they become your strengths.

—Knute Rockne

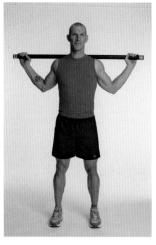 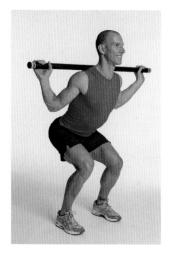 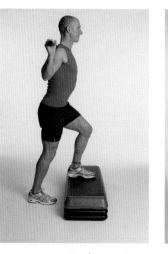

Basic Squat

Front Step-Up (one side at a time)

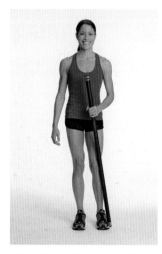 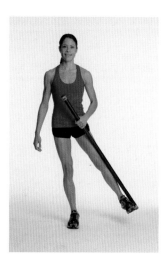 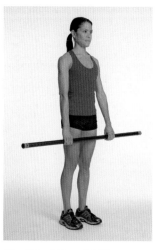 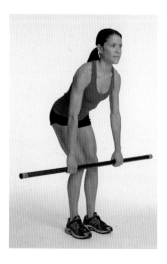

Standing Side Leg Lift

Modified Dead Lift

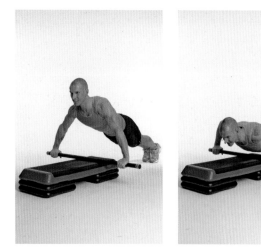 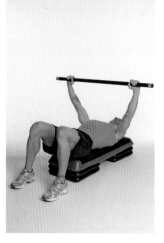 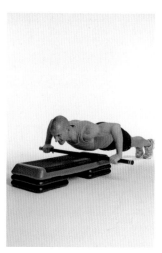

Straight-Arm Plank (15–30 seconds; remember: kneeling is an option)

Chest Press

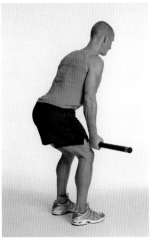
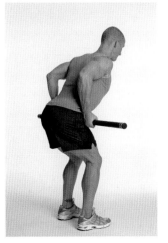

Narrow-Grip Bent-Over Row

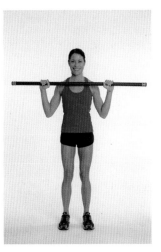

Shoulder Press

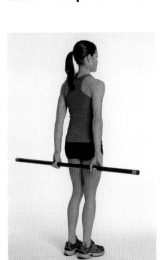
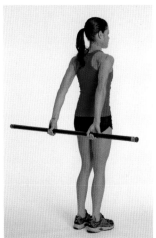

Rear Shoulder Extension

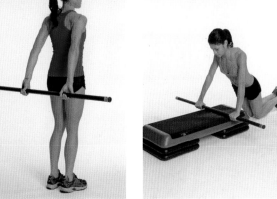

Straight-Arm Plank (15–30 seconds; remember: kneeling is an option)

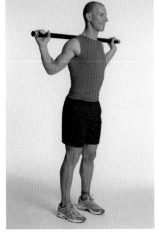
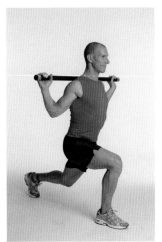

Forward Lunge (alternating legs; use the bar for balance if necessary)

If I had six hours to chop down a tree, I'd spend the first four hours sharpening an axe.

—Abraham Lincoln

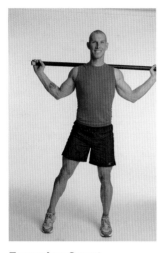 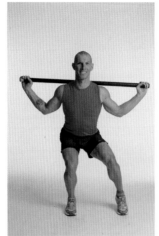 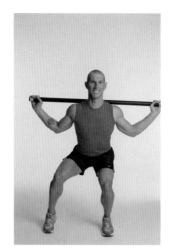

Frowning Squat

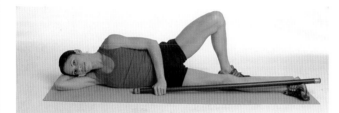

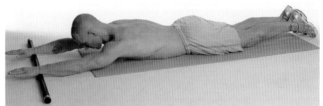

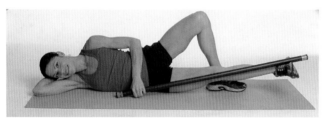

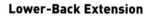

Side-Lying Inner-Thigh Lift

Lower-Back Extension

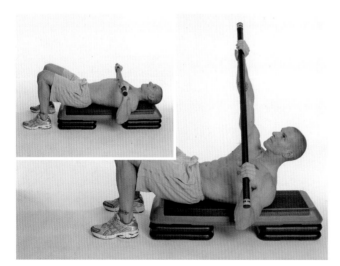

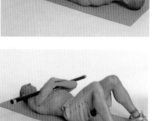 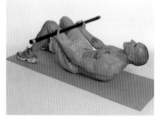

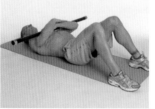 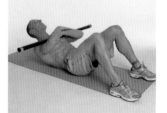

Abdominal Crunch with Single-Arm Chest Press

Abdominal Crunch (with the bar either on your hips or cradled across your chest)

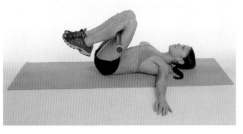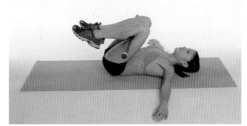

Reverse Crunch with Bar Behind Knees

Full Body—Beginner 3

Time: 20–40 minutes

Props: Body Bar, platform

Drill: Do 15 reps of each exercise. For single-sided exercises, do a full set on each side. If you make it through this circuit and feel like you are ready to take it to the next level, go through the circuit twice or do two sets of each exercise before moving on to the next.

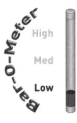

Basic Squat

Forward Lunge (one side at a time)

Shoulder Press

Wide-Grip Bent-Over Row

Reverse Lunge (alternating sides; use the bar for balance if necessary)

Smiley Squat

Rear Shoulder Extension

Squat with Shoulder Press

Push-Up

Shoulder External Rotation

Bridge

Modified Roll Down

Abdominal Crunch with Single-Arm Chest Press

Side Crunch

Lower-Back Extension

Straight-Arm Plank (20–30 seconds; remember: kneeling is an option)

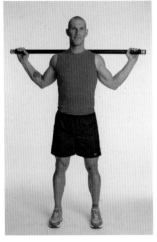 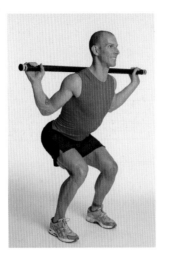 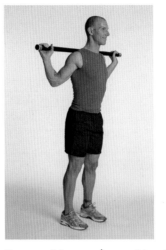 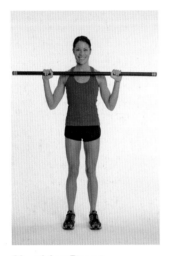

Basic Squat

Forward Lunge (one side at a time)

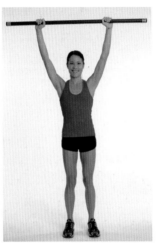 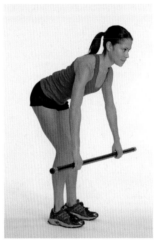 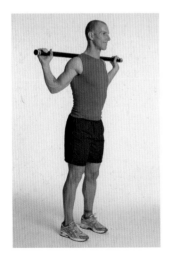 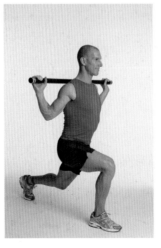

Shoulder Press

Wide-Grip Bent-Over Row

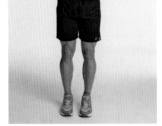 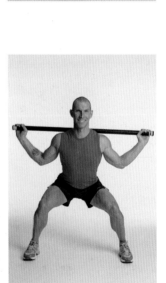

Reverse Lunge (alternating sides; use the bar for balance if necessary)

Smiley Squat

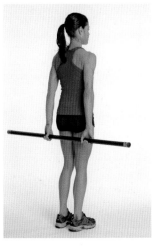
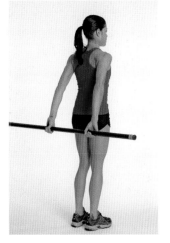

Rear Shoulder Extension

Motivation gets you going.
Discipline keeps you going.

—Jim Ryan

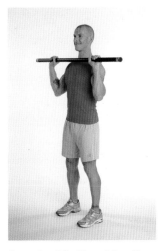
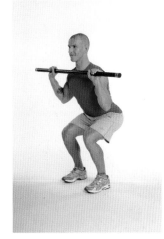

Squat with Shoulder Press

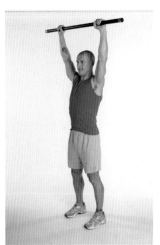
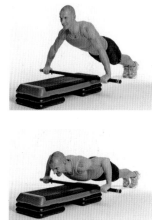

Push-Up

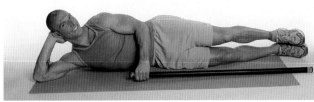
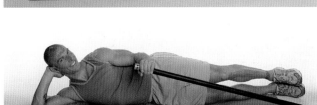

Shoulder External Rotation

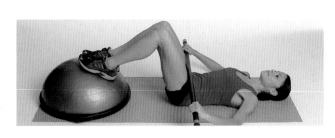
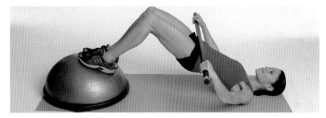

Bridge

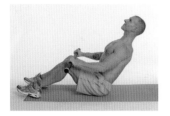
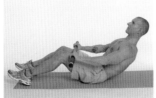
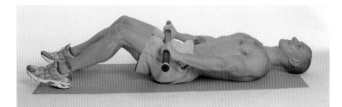

Modified Roll Down

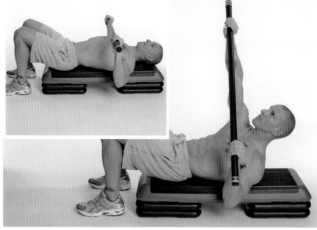

Abdominal Crunch with Single-Arm Chest Press

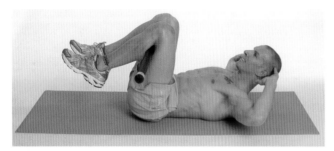

Side Crunch

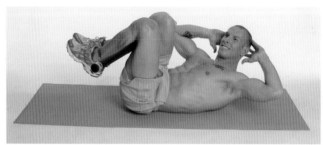

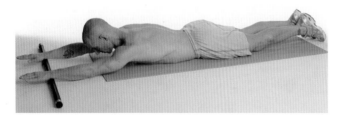
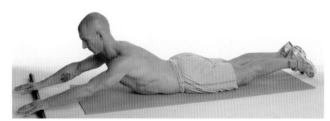

Lower-Back Extension

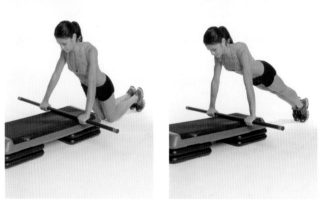

Straight-Arm Plank (20–30 seconds; remember: kneeling is an option)

Full Body—Intermediate

Time: 25–50 minutes

Props: Body Bar, platform

Drill: Do 15–20 reps of each exercise. For single-sided exercises, do a full set on each side. If you make it through this circuit and feel like you are ready to take it to the next level, go through the circuit twice or do two sets of each exercise before moving on to the next.

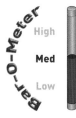

Straight-Arm Plank (30–60 seconds)

Basic Squat with Rotation (16–20 squats)

Single-Arm Narrow-Grip Bent-Over Row

Side Lunge (alternating legs; use the bar for balance if necessary)

Push-Up

Single-Arm Rear Deltoid Fly (rest one end of the bar on the floor if necessary)

Reverse Lunge with Biceps Curl (alternating legs)

Squat with Shoulder Press and Rotation (16–20 squats)

Modified Single-Leg Dead Lift

Pendulum (alternating sides)

Basic Lunge with Rotation

Single-Arm Chest Press

Kayaker

Roll Down

Plank with Hip Extension (alternating legs)

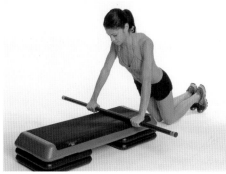
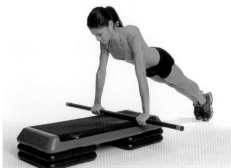

Straight-Arm Plank (30–60 seconds)

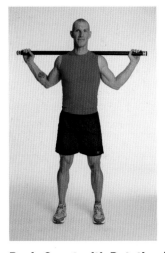
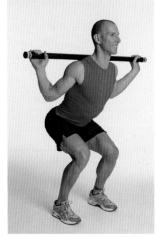
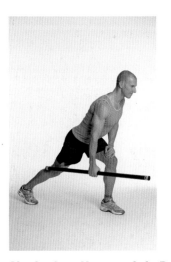

Basic Squat with Rotation (16–20 squats)

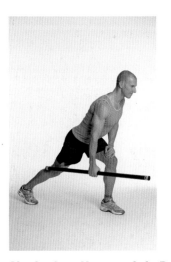
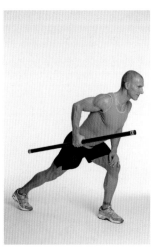

Single-Arm Narrow-Grip Bent-Over Row

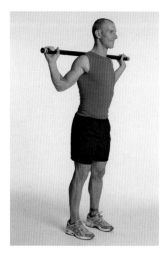
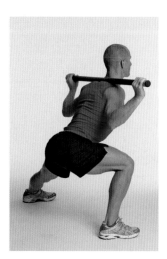

Side Lunge (alternating legs; use the bar for balance if necessary)

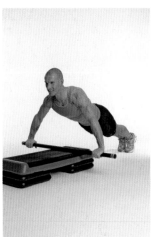
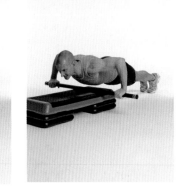

Push-Up

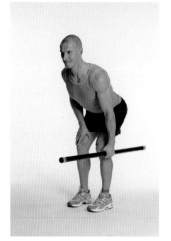
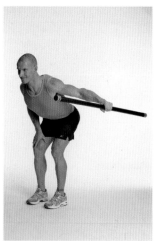

Single-Arm Rear Deltoid Fly (rest one end of the bar on the floor if necessary)

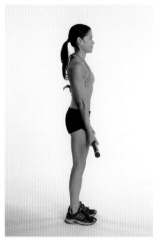

**Reverse Lunge with Biceps Curl
(alternating legs)**

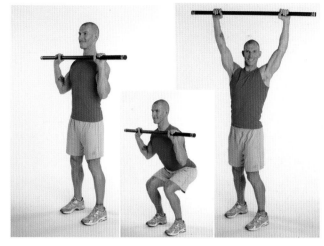

**Squat with Shoulder Press and Rotation
(16–20 squats)**

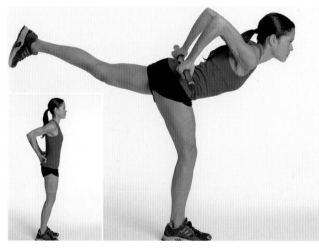

Modified Single-Leg Dead Lift

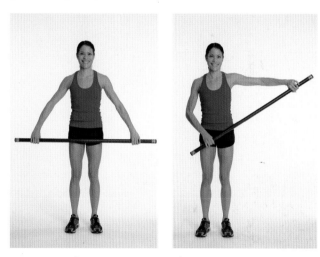

Pendulum (alternating sides)

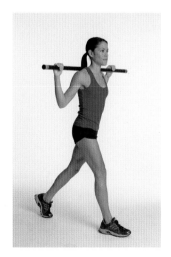
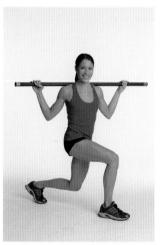

**Basic Lunge with
Rotation**

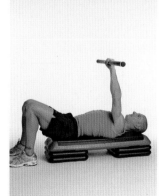
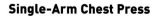
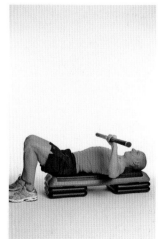

Single-Arm Chest Press

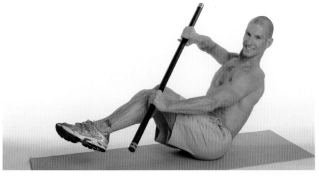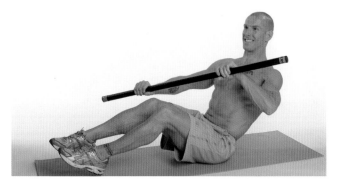

Kayaker

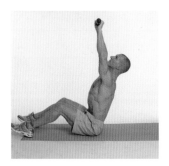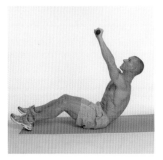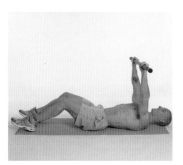

Roll Down

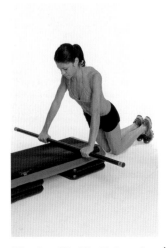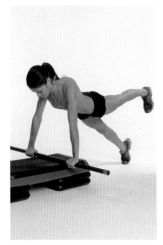

Plank with Hip Extension (alternating legs)

Full Body—Intermediate–Advanced 1

Time: 25–50 minutes

Props: Body Bar, platform

Drill: Do 15–20 reps of each exercise, unless otherwise noted. For single-sided exercises, do a full set on each side. If you make it through this circuit and feel like you are ready to take it to the next level, go through the circuit twice or do two sets of each exercise before moving on to the next.

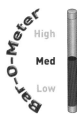

Basic Squat with Rotation and Knee Lift

Single-Leg Squat

Push-Up

Single-Arm Chest Fly

Lunge with Rear Leg Elevation

Modified Single-Leg Dead Lift

Wide-Grip Bent-Over Row

Single-Arm Narrow-Grip Bent-Over Row

Side Lunge with Pendulum

Rainbow Squat (16–20 squats)

Clean-and-Press with Rotation

Curtsy Lunge with Upright Row (with optional kick)

Single-Arm Rear Deltoid Fly

Narrow-Grip Bent-Over Row

Single-Arm Chest Press

Chest Press with Pullover Arc

Bridge

Static Bridge with Leg Extension (hold for 20–30 seconds)

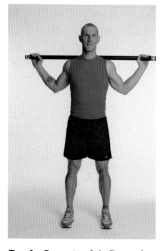 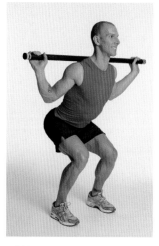 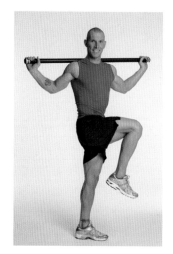

Basic Squat with Rotation and Knee lift

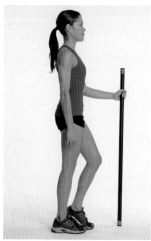 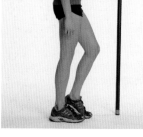 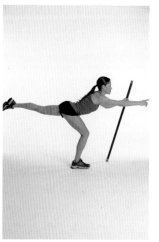 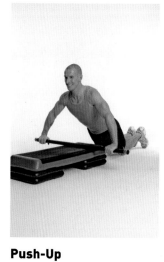 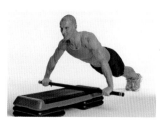 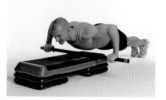

Single-Leg Squat

Push-Up

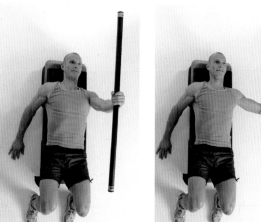 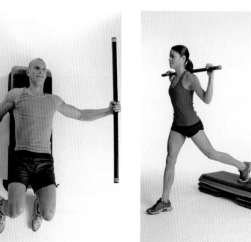 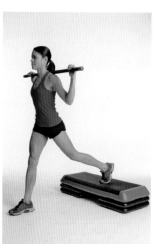

Single-Arm Chest Fly

Lunge with Rear Leg Elevation

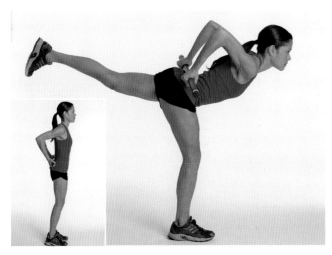

Modified Single-Leg Dead Lift

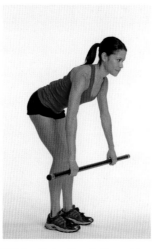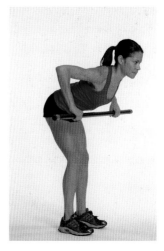

Wide-Grip Bent-Over Row

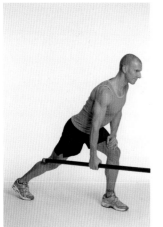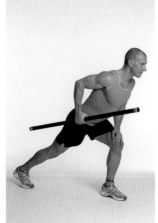

Single-Arm Narrow-Grip Bent-Over Row

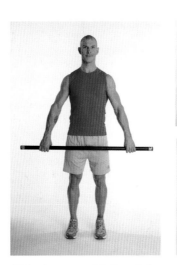

Side Lunge with Pendulum

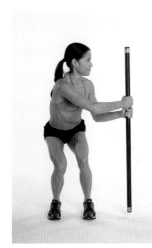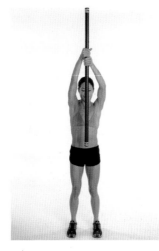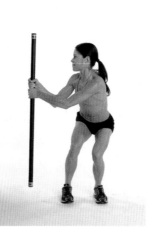

Rainbow Squat (16–20 squats)

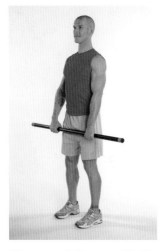 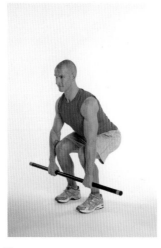 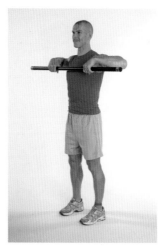 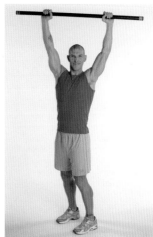

Clean-and-Press with Rotation

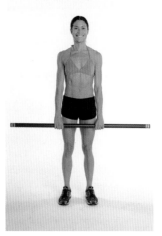 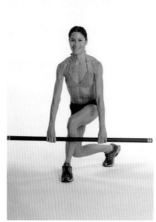 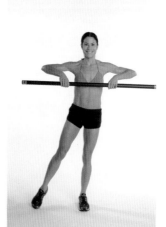 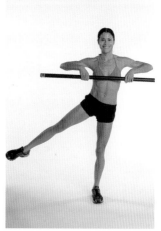

Curtsy Lunge with Upright Row

(with optional kick)

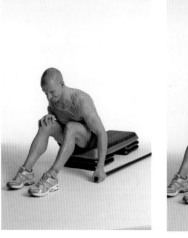 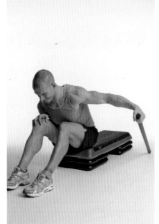

Single-Arm Rear Deltoid Fly

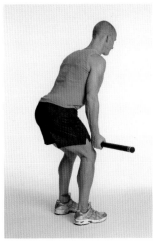 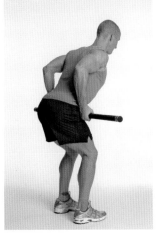

Narrow-Grip Bent-Over Row

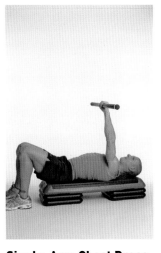 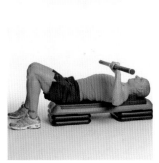

Single-Arm Chest Press

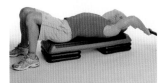

Chest Press with Pullover Arc

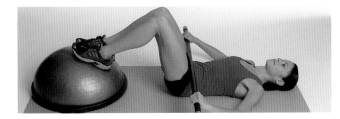

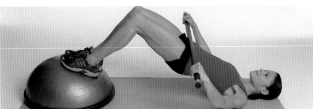

Bridge

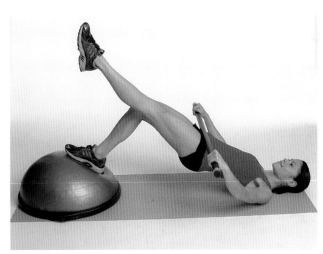

Static Bridge with Leg Extension (hold for 20–30 seconds)

Time: 10, 20, or 30 minutes

Props: Body Bar, platform

Drill: Do 15–20 reps of each exercise, unless otherwise noted. For single-sided exercises, do a full set on each side. Complete the full circuit between one and three times, depending on the amount of time you have and the type of challenge you are looking for. Going through this circuit once will take you about 10 minutes. You can also complement this workout with one of the core workouts.

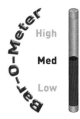

Squat Thrust

Push-Up

Single-Leg Squat

Roll Down

Reverse Lunge with Single-Arm Press

Single-Arm Wide-Grip Bent-Over Row

Split Squat Jump on a Platform (10–12 each side)

Kayaker

Squat with Shoulder Press and Rotation

Push-Up

Front-to-Back Lunge with Biceps Curl

Running Plank

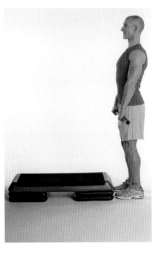 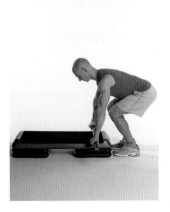 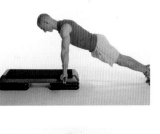 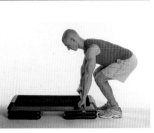 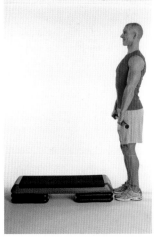

Squat Thrust

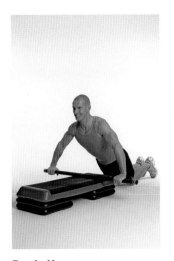 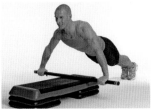 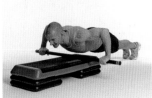 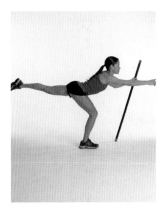

Push-Up

Single-Leg Squat

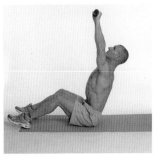 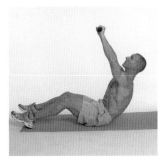 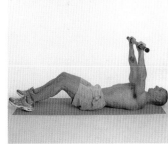

Roll Down

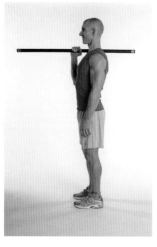 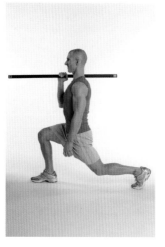 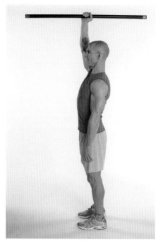 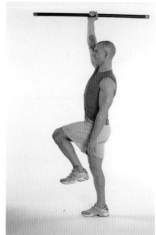

Reverse Lunge with Single-Arm Press

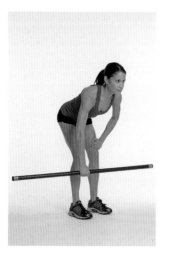 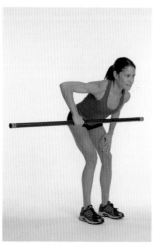

Single-Arm Wide-Grip Bent-Over Row

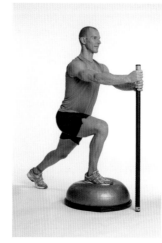

Split Squat Jump on a Platform

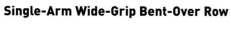
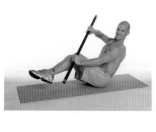
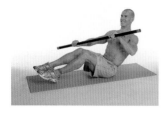

Kayaker

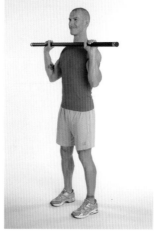

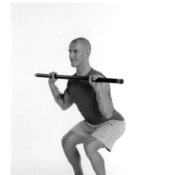 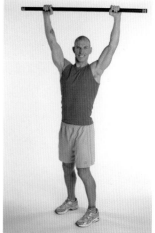

Squat with Shoulder Press and Rotation

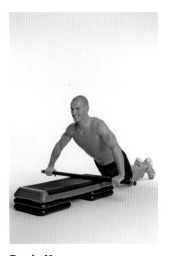 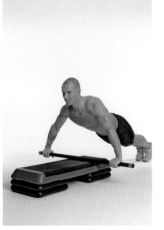 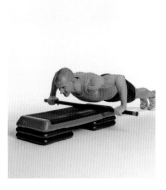

Push-Up

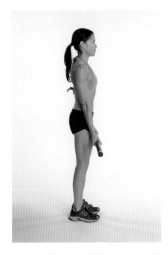 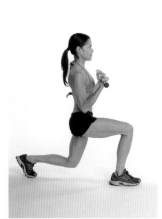 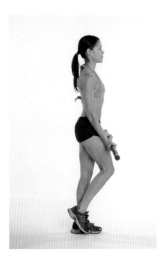 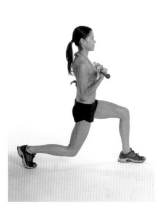

Front-to-Back Lunge with Biceps Curl

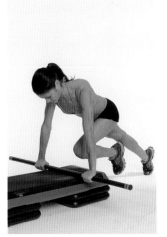 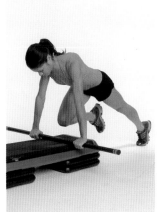

Running Plank

Full Body with Anaerobic Infusion—Advanced 1

> **Time:** 25–50 minutes
>
> **Props:** Body Bar, platform
>
> **Drill:** Do 15–20 reps of each exercise. For single-sided exercises, do a full set on each side.

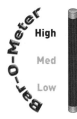

Clean-and-Press to Calf Raise

Single-Arm Row with Knee Lift

Ultimate Full-Body Combo

Modified Single-Leg Dead Lift with Narrow-Grip Row

Hot Feet (30–45 seconds)

1–2-minute recovery

Rainbow Squat (16–20 squats)

Crab Walk (take 3 steps to each side)

Dead Lift to Pendulum (one side at a time)

Curtsy Lunge with Upright Row (16–20 upright rows)

Lateral Leap (30–45 seconds)

1–2-minute recovery

Squat Thrust Push-Up

Reverse Lunge with Single-Arm Press

Stir the Pot and Squat (stir 8–10 times in each direction)

Front-to-Back Lunge with Biceps Curl

Slalom

1–2-minute recovery

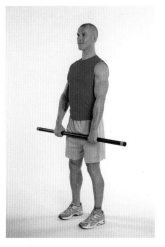 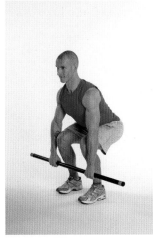 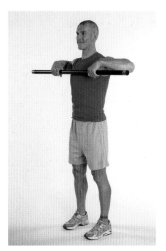 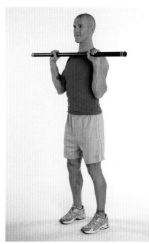

Clean-and-Press to Calf Raise

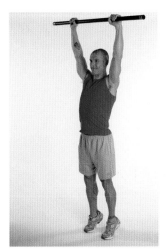 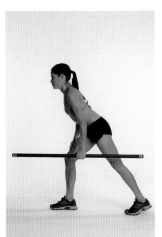 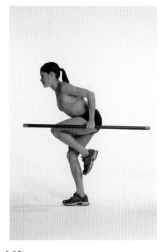

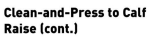

Clean-and-Press to Calf Raise (cont.)

Single-Arm Row with Knee Lift

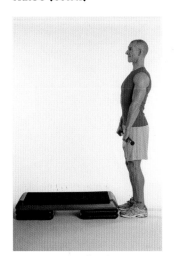

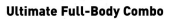

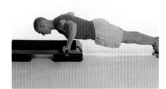

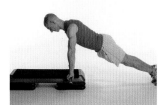 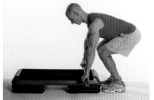

Ultimate Full-Body Combo

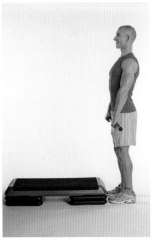 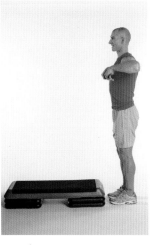 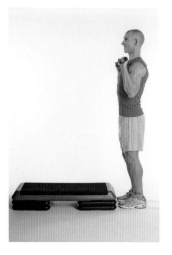 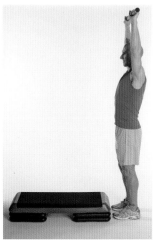

Ultimate Full-Body Combo (cont.)

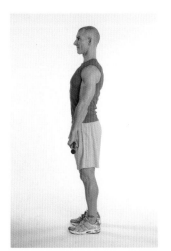 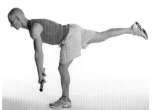 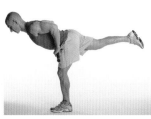 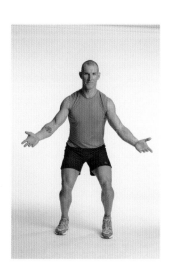 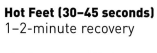

Modified Single-Leg Dead Lift with Narrow-Grip Row

Hot Feet (30–45 seconds)
1–2-minute recovery

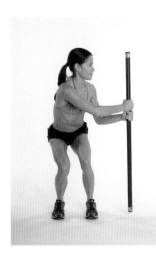 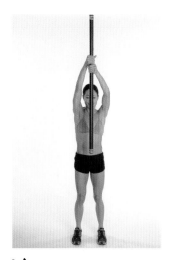 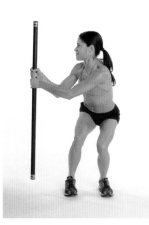

Rainbow Squat (16–20 squats)

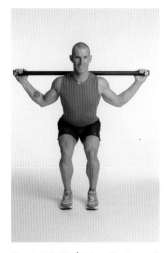 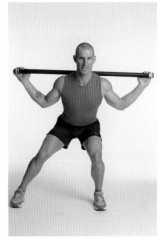 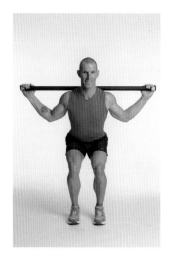

Crab Walk (take 3 steps to each side)

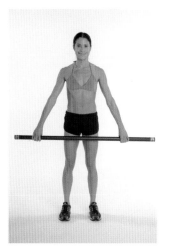 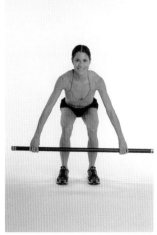 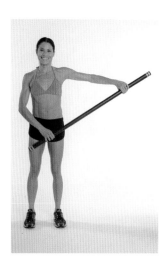

Dead Lift to Pendulum (one side at a time)

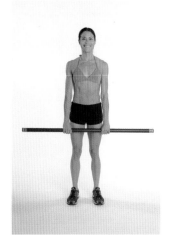 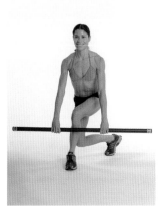 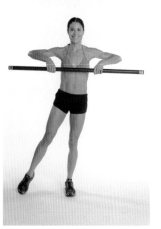

Curtsy Lunge with Upright Row (16–20 upright rows)

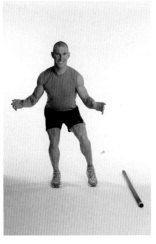 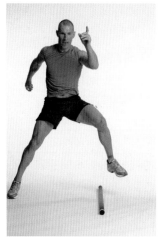 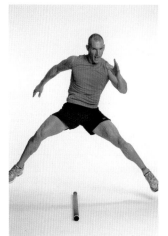 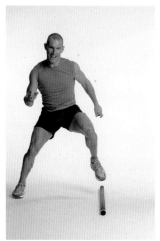

Lateral Leap (30–45 seconds)
1–2-minute recovery

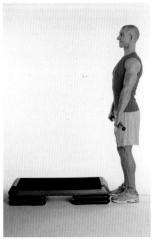 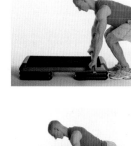 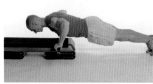 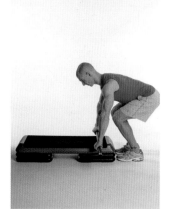
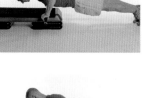

Squat Thrust Push-Up

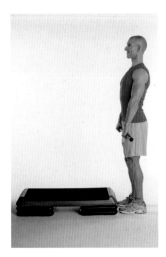 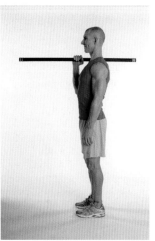 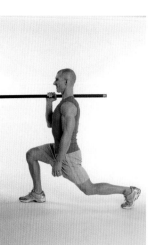 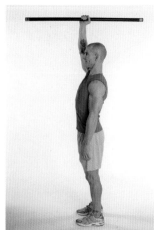

**Squat Thrust Push-Up
(cont.)**　　　　**Reverse Lunge with Single-Arm Press**

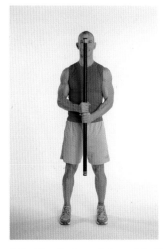 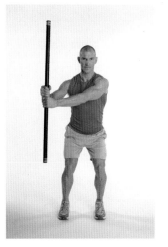 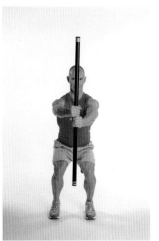 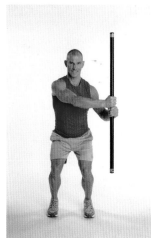

Stir the Pot and Squat (stir 8–10 times in each direction)

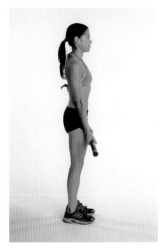 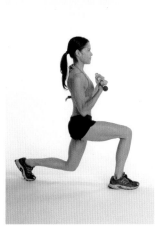 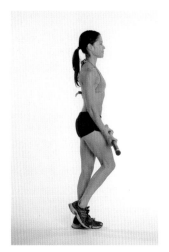 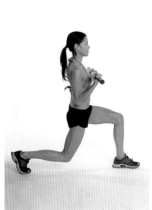

Front-to-Back Lunge with Biceps Curl

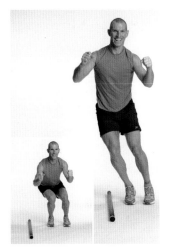 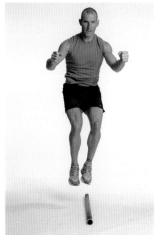 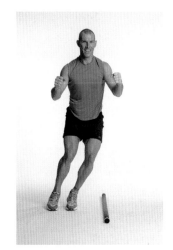 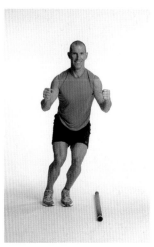

Slalom
1–2-minute recovery

Full Body with Anaerobic Infusion—Advanced 2

Time: 30–60 minutes

Props: Body Bar, platform

Drill: Do 15–20 reps of each exercise. For single-sided exercises, do a full set on each side.

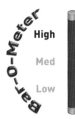

Basic Squat

Shoulder Press

Wide-Grip Bent-Over Row

Lunge with Rear Leg Elevation

Lateral Leap (20–30 seconds)

Hot Feet (20–30 seconds)

Split Squat Jump (20–30 seconds)

1–2-minute recovery

Single-Leg Squat

Single-Arm Rear Deltoid Fly

Push-Up

Squat with Shoulder Press and Rotation (16–20 squats)

Lateral Leap (20–30 seconds)

Hot Feet (20–30 seconds)

Split Squat Jump (20–30 seconds)

1–2-minute recovery

Clean-and-Press

Pendulum

Single-Arm Narrow-Grip Bent-Over Row

Reverse Lunge with Biceps Curl (alternating sides)

Lateral Leap (20–30 seconds)

Hot Feet (20–30 seconds)

Split Squat Jump (20–30 seconds)

1–2-minute recovery

Rainbow Squat (16–20 squats)

Push-Up

Running Plank

Bridge

Lateral Leap (20–30 seconds)

Hot Feet (20–30 seconds)

Split Squat Jump (20–30 seconds)

1–2-minute recovery

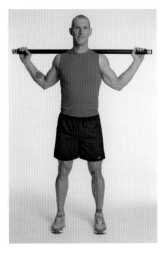 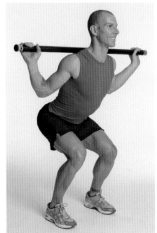 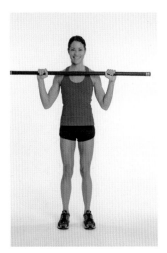 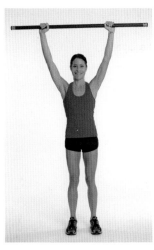

Basic Squat   **Shoulder Press**

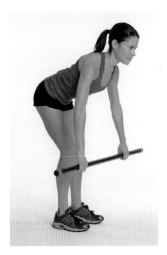 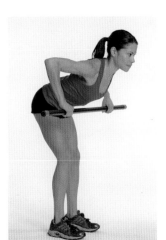 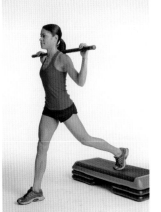 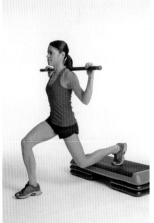

Wide-Grip Bent-Over Row   **Lunge with Rear Leg Elevation**

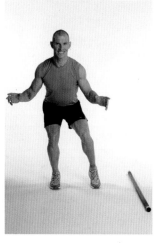 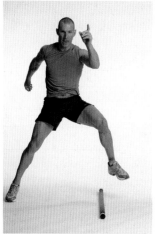 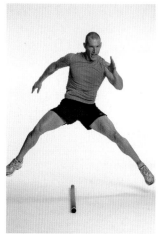 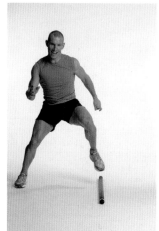

Lateral Leap (20–30 seconds)

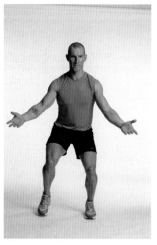 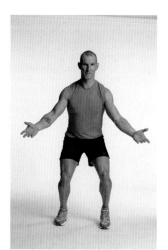 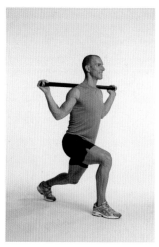

Hot Feet (20–30 seconds)

Split Squat Jump (20–30 seconds)

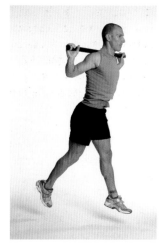 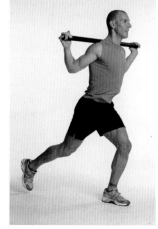 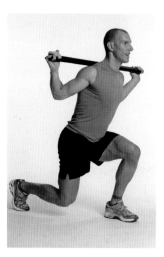

Split Squat Jump (20–30 seconds) cont.
1–2-minute recovery

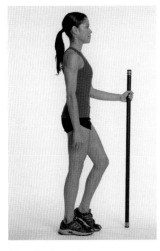

Single-Leg Squat

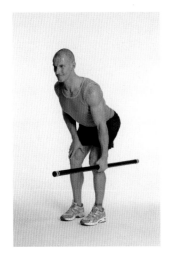

Single-Arm Rear Deltoid Fly

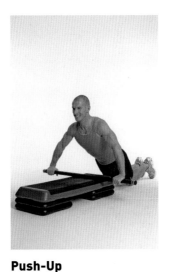

Push-Up

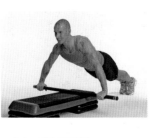

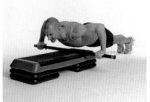

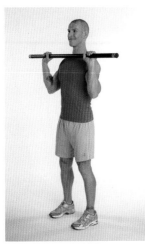

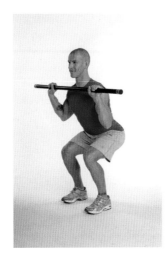

**Squat with Shoulder Press and Rotation
(16–20 squats)**

Repeat the Lateral Leap, Hot Feet, and Split Squat Jump exercises for 20–30 seconds each. Take 1–2 minutes to catch your breath and recover before moving on.

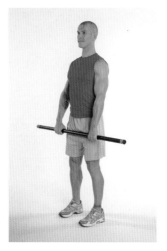 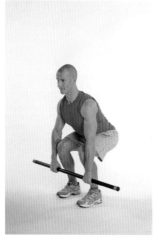 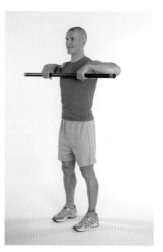 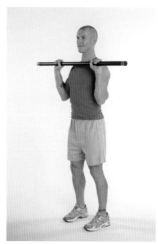

Clean-and-Press

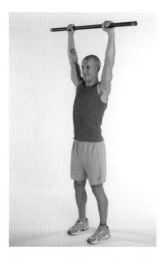 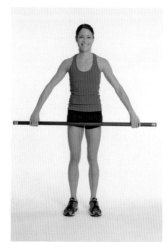 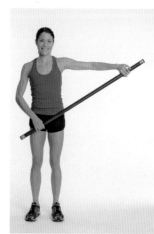

Clean-and-Press (cont.)   **Pendulum**

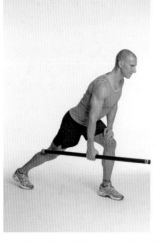 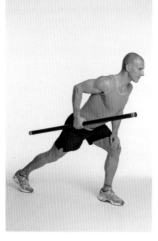 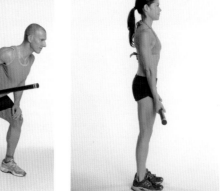

Single-Arm Narrow-Grip Bent-Over Row   **Reverse Lunge with Biceps Curl (alternating sides)**

Repeat the Lateral Leap, Hot Feet, and Split Squat Jump exercises for 20–30 seconds each. Take 1–2 minutes to catch your breath and recover before moving on.

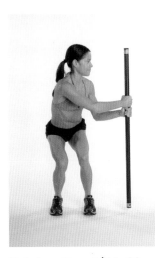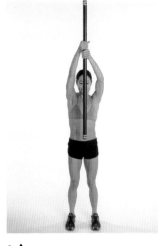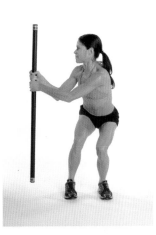

Rainbow Squat (16–20 squats)

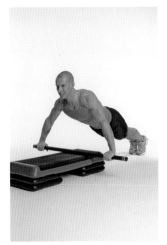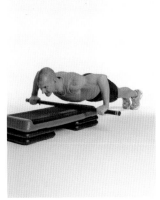

Push-Up

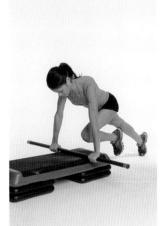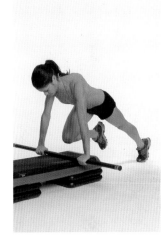

Running Plank

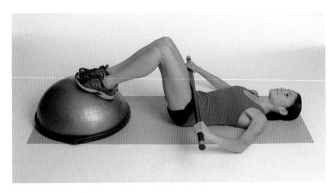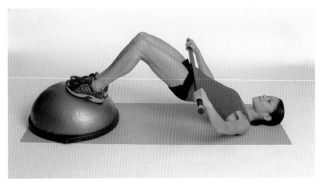

Bridge

Repeat the Lateral Leap, Hot Feet, and Split Squat Jump exercises for 20–30 seconds each. Take 1–2 minutes to catch your breath and recover before moving on.

Core—Beginner

Time: 5–10 minutes

Props: Body Bar, platform

Drill: Do 10–15 reps of each exercise. For single-sided exercises, do a full set on each side. Go through this circuit once or twice.

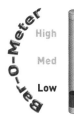

Straight-Arm Plank

Bridge

Side Crunch

Reverse Crunch

Abdominal Crunch (with the bar either on your hips or cradled across your chest)

Lower-Back Extension

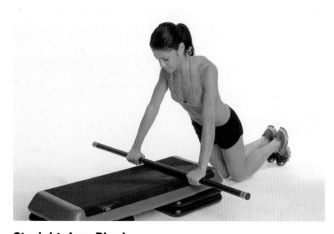

Straight-Arm Plank

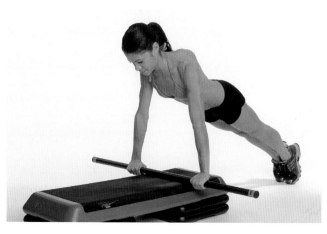

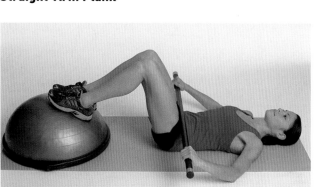

Bridge

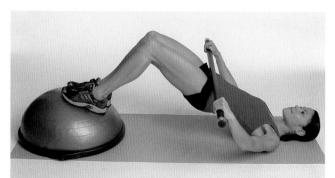

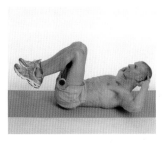 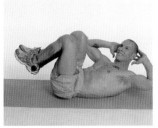 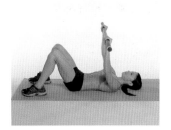 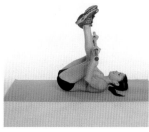

Side Crunch   **Reverse Crunch**

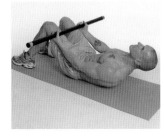 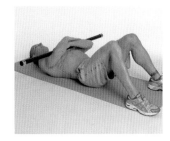 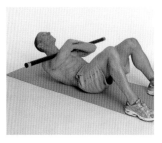

Abdominal Crunch (with the bar either on your hips or cradled across your chest)

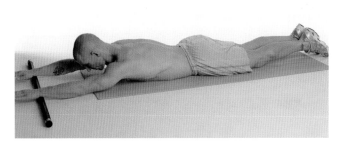 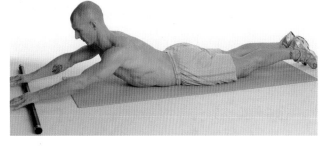

Lower-Back Extension

Core—Intermediate—Advanced

Time: 10–20 minutes

Props: Body Bar, platform (try a Bosu for a supercharged experience)

Drill: Do 15–25 reps of each exercise. For single-sided exercises, do a full set on each side. Go through this circuit once or twice.

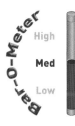

Straight-Arm Plank (hold for 30–60 seconds)

Bicycle Crunch

Abdominal Crunch with Single-Arm Chest Press

Reverse Crunch with Bar Behind Knees

Running Plank

Lower-Back Extension

Abdominal Crunch

Kayaker

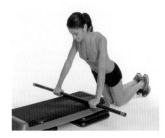 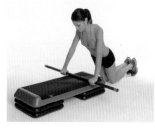 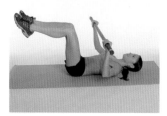 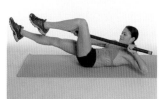

Straight-Arm Plank (hold for 30–60 seconds) **Bicycle Crunch**

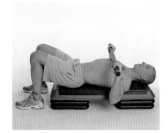 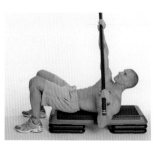 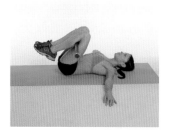 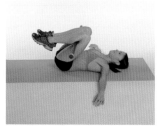

Abdominal Crunch with Single-Arm Chest Press **Reverse Crunch with Bar Behind Knees**

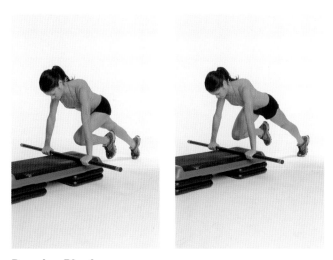

Running Plank

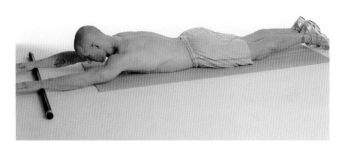 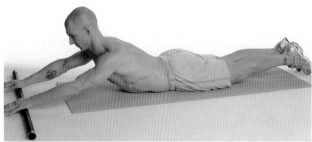

Lower-Back Extension

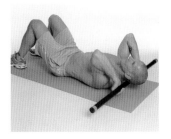 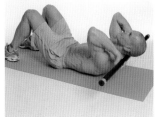

Abdominal Crunch

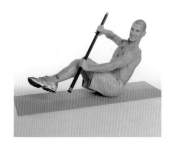 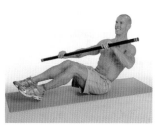

Kayaker

Core—Advanced

Time: 10–20 minutes

Props: Body Bar, platform (try a Bosu for a supercharged experience)

Drill: Do 15–25 reps of each exercise. For single-sided exercises, do a full set on each side. Go through this circuit once or twice.

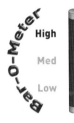

Bar-O-Meter High / Med / Low

Straight-Arm Plank

Bicycle Crunch

Reverse Crunch

Side Crunch

Plank with Hip Extension

Roll Down

Full-Body Crunch

Hip Crossover

Static Bridge with Leg Extension

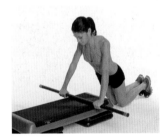
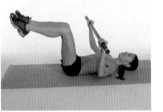

Straight-Arm Plank

Bicycle Crunch

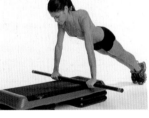
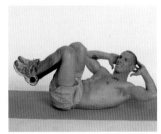

Reverse Crunch

Side Crunch

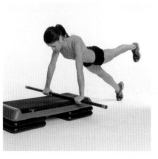 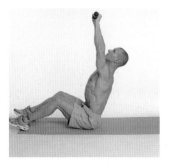 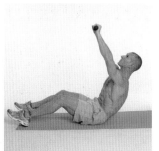 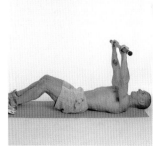

Plank with Hip Extension **Roll Down**

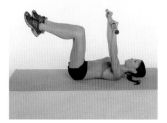 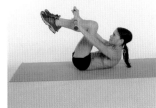 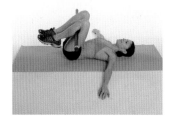 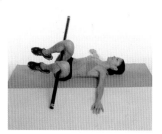

Full-Body Crunch **Hip Crossover**

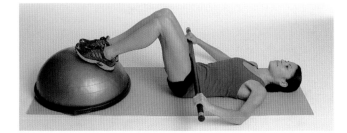

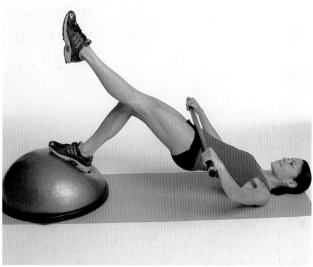

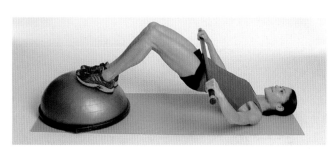

Static Bridge with Leg Extension

Success is sweet, but usually has
the scent of sweat about it.

—Anonymous

The Home Stretch

To develop and maintain your flexibility, it is imperative that you practice it, as you practice any other part of your fitness routine (cardio, strength, balance). It is just as important. Besides, it just feels so good. It is like the heavenly reward after a challenging workout.

Here are a few sample remedies for stretching the most common tight spots. Do not feel limited to the stretches we describe. You are at liberty to do any types of stretches you prefer as long as you know what you are doing. Stretching gone wrong is more common than you think. Be as careful with stretching as you are with any other type of physical activity.

Wonder Bar

Wondering . . . when the best time to stretch is? We recommend stretching after a workout, when your body is most supple. Theoretically, you are at greater risk of injury otherwise.

If you want to learn more about stretching, we recommend taking a look at a book by a great friend and mentor, Jay Blahnik, called *Full-Body Flexibility*. It is interesting and informative and will guide you through a ton of brilliant stretches (see www.jayblahnik.com).

The Stretches

The Tight Spot: Hamstrings

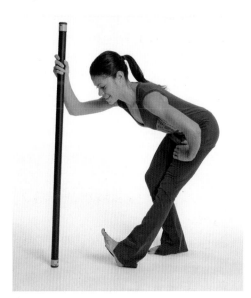

Did you know that when we stretch, we are actually damaging our muscles in the minutest of ways? Not to worry, this damage repairs itself amazingly, in a more flexible way. (We learned this from Jay!)

The Prescription: Single-Leg Forward Bend

The Directions: Bring one foot forward, keeping your weight over the ankle of your back foot. With your back flat and your forward leg straight, bend your back knee and hinge at the hips until you feel the stretch in the hamstring of the front leg. Hold for 15 to 45 seconds.

The Tight Spot: Quadriceps

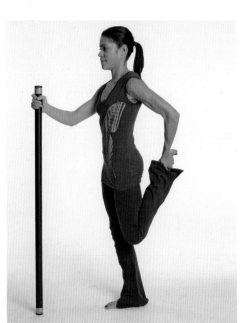

The Prescription: Standing Quadriceps Stretch

The Directions: Begin standing, holding the Body Bar vertically in one hand for balance if necessary. Grasp the opposite foot in your hand and pull your heel toward your gluteals until you feel a stretch in your quadriceps. Hold for 15 to 45 seconds.

The Tight Spot: Hip Flexor

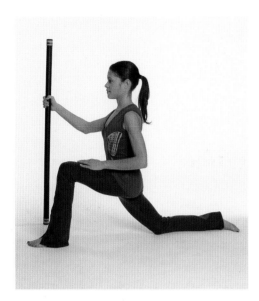

The Prescription: Deep Lunge

The Directions: In a deep lunge, with your back knee resting on the floor, hold the Body Bar vertically with the hand on the side of your back leg for balance if necessary. Push through your hip as you lift through your chest until you feel the stretch at the top of your back leg into the region of your abs. Hold for 15 to 45 seconds.

The Tight Spot: Gluteals

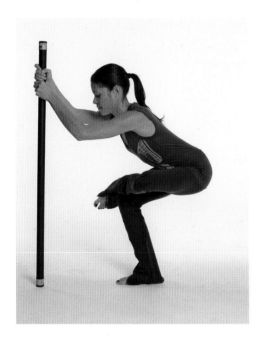

The Prescription: Standing Ankle-to-Knee Stretch

The Directions: Begin standing, holding the Body Bar vertically in both hands for balance. Bring one ankle across the opposite knee. Keeping your back flat, bend your standing leg and push your hips back and the top of the bar away from you until you feel the stretch in the gluteals of the crossed leg. Hold for 15 to 45 seconds. If you are having trouble doing this stretch standing, try it seated.

The Tight Spot: Calves

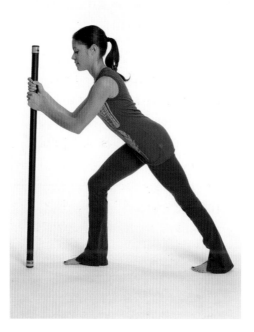

The Prescription: Calf Stretch from Lunge

The Directions: Begin in a lunge position, holding the Body Bar vertically in one or both hands for balance and to support your upper-body weight. Push your back heel into the floor as you hinge forward, keeping your body in a straight line from the top of your head down to your heel. You should feel this stretch in the calf of your back leg. Hold for 15 to 45 seconds.

"Knead" a massage? As a gesture of gratitude, the Body Bar is happy to offer you a special treat. Place the Body Bar on the floor and roll your foot over it. Put as much weight on the bar as feels comfortable to you. Take a deep breath and relax.

The Tight Spot: Chest

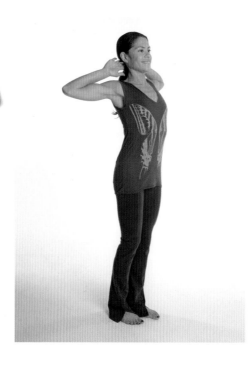

The Prescription: Chest Stretch

The Directions: With your fingertips lightly touching the back of your head, extend both elbows directly out to the sides. Reach back with your elbows, squeezing your shoulder blades together. You should feel the stretch through your chest and the front of your shoulders. Imagine trying to touch your elbows behind your back. Keep your neck long. Hold for a few seconds, release, and repeat 10 to 15 times.

The Tight Spot: Back

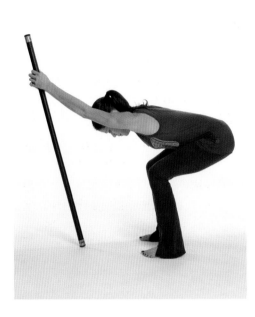

The Prescription: Standing Lat Stretch

The Directions: Begin standing, holding the Body Bar vertically in both hands approximately 10 to 12 inches in front of you. Sit back into a squat as you push the top of the bar away in an angle across your body. Push your hips away from the bar. You should feel the stretch down the side of your back. Hold for 15 to 45 seconds.

The Tight Spot: Lower Back

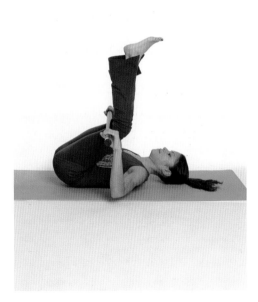

The Prescription: Lower-Back Roll

The Directions: Lie on your back, grasping the Body Bar with a wide grip behind your knees. Pull the bar toward you until your hips and lower back roll off the floor. Hold for a moment, release, and repeat. You can also try rolling your hips in a circular motion.

Resources

So, now you want to buy a Body Bar or two. Admit it, don't be bashful, you are hooked. We are happy to have whetted your appetite. We are here to satisfy your new vice—a surprisingly healthy one at that. The following Web sites can all lead you to Body Bar proprietorship and more.

www.bodybars.com
This is the official Body Bar site. You can purchase you bar (or bars) on this site, as well as a number of Body Bar workout DVDs.

www.performbetter.com
www.power-systems.com
Both of the sites listed above carry Body Bars and are incredible resources for fitness equipment in general.

For the stretch book mentioned earlier in this book, please visit www.jahblahnik.com.

For a BOSU Balance Trainer and other associated training DVDs and videos, see www.bosu.com.

For information and purchase of our favorite sports drink, see www.amino-vital.com.

Check with your local gym to see if they offer group fitness classes using Body Bars. Group classes are a great way to introduce yourself and get used to some of the moves using Body Bars in a safe and guided environment.

Do you have any questions and/or comments, etc.? Please contact us at www.greggcook.com.

Index

With Thanks:

We are eternally grateful for the opportunity to share a bit of our-selves, and what we believe may help make your life better, even if just by an infinitesimal bit. We thank you for your time (we know how limited it can seem) and ask that if in fact taking some of the things you have learned from us in this book has brought you some positive change in your life, in return you will pay it forward.

With humble (and healthy) hearts, love, and respect,
Gregg and Fatima

Be in touch. See www.greggcook.com

With Special Thanks:

To God, our moms and dads, family and friends, Julie Trelstad, Abby Rabinowitz, Sherry Catlin, Harry and Phillip, and our mentors: Douglas Brooks and Candice Copeland Brooks, and Jay Blahnik. We'd also like to thank Equinox for everything throughout the years.